Virility Factor

Masculinity Through Testosterone,
The Male Sex Hormone

by Robert Bahr

FACTOR PRESS

6920 Airport Boulevard
#117-100
Mobile, Alabama 36608
U.S.A.

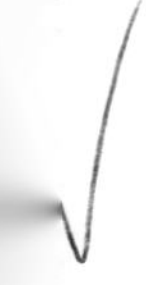

First edition published by G. P. Putnam's Sons, New York

ISBN 0-9626531-1-X

To Those Who Helped

This book is about a hormone. That, by definition, makes it a fascinating subject, for there is nothing more exciting in medicine than these incredibly powerful substances and the awesome influences they wield over the body. What's more, they comprise probably the fastest-growing medical field today, for both researchers and practitioners realize that the hormones and the endocrine glands that secrete them hold many more keys to illness and health than we have ever guessed.

That enthusiasm for endocrinology poses the first problem in preparing a book of this sort: Of the new research being published continuously in all areas of the field, which are the soundest, most widely held interpretations of the findings?

Without the help of the specialists themselves, no writer can hope to answer that. In receiving information, detailed criticism, and recommendations from several of the nation's most eminent endocrinologists, I have been particularly fortunate. My gratitude to:

Herbert Kupperman, MD, PhD, New York City.

Mortimer B. Lipsett, MD, Director, The Cancer Center, Inc., Cincinnati, Ohio.

Norman Orentreich, MD, and J. H. Vogelman, MD, The Orentreich Medical Group, New York City.

Charles T. Kuntzleman, PhD, Director, Y-Fitness Finders, Spring Arbor, Michigan.

Thanks also to Daniel S. Rogers of the National Institute of Health's Gerontology Research Center at the Baltimore City Hospitals, and to the Endocrine Society and the Pharmaceutical Information Bureau for the help and cooperation of their spokesmen.

I'm particularly grateful to editor Edward T. Chase for his enthusiastic support and guidance throughout the project.

Assisting in the research and manuscript preparation were Carol Nippert, Barbara Yobst, E. C. Carver, Jr., Barbara Erich, and Alice Bahr.

A second problem in writing a book like this is the subject matter's controversial nature. Many experts see a thing one way and have an assortment of studies to support their views. Yet an equally large group of equally respected authorities, also with supporting data, hold with great tenacity to a different, and perhaps even conflicting, view. That is when the writer himself, after studying the literature and conducting his interviews, must decide for himself.

Regardless of which side of the fence he finally stands on, the writer will obviously receive frowns from those who hold opposing views. Let it be clarified that the interpretations, where required, are mine and not necessarily those of the people without whose help this book would have been far more difficult to write.

Contents

Introduction

Countless books and articles have discussed for the lay reader the fascinating subject of female endocrinology and hormones. But the endocrinology of the male and the effect inadequate testosterone levels may produce in him have been virtually ignored in popular writing. When it is discussed at all, it is shrouded in myth and superstition. Robert Bahr's book makes an essential contribution to a subject as basic to every man as his self-image and his capacity to function as a man.

The endocrine-deficient male has been neglected with respect to appropriate therapy, a fact that Mr. Bahr has well emphasized. A male wears his gonads externally; he is open to inspection and ridicule when he deviates from the norm. When these gonads do not measure up to what the normal standard would be, the male may be affected by this, as reflected in his mental attitude and lack of normal aggressiveness.

The lack of masculine aggressiveness may be a measure of a male's testosterone deficiency. The dominant pecking order in the fowl, as well as the dominant role of the male in animals that live in large groups, particularly the monkey, appear to be related to testosterone levels. When these levels are adequate, the normal male response is seen. In fact, increased testosterone levels above the norm occur in the dominant male who is the leader of the pack. When the male hormone is deficient, at least in the animal kingdom, there is a tendency for these males to accept a passive role. The same applies to the human male. When testosterone levels are inadequate, physical debilitation associated with poor muscular development may occur, and changes in personality may be seen. It is for this reason that wise and early implementation of appropriate therapy would be helpful in preventing some disastrous psychological aberrations from taking place in the male.

It is equally important to know that penile vigor and

masculinity are measures of one's hormonal levels, although this may vary, depending upon the responsiveness of one's tissues and organs to testosterone. In other words, in two men with exactly the same testosterone level, one may have a large penis and one may have a relatively small one, due to the fact that the end organ, namely the penis, is more refractory, or not responsive to the action of his own inwardly produced hormones. Another example of this, of course, is female breast development. Two women may have essentially the same amount of female sex hormones, yet their breast sizes vary greatly, depending upon the responsiveness of the tissue, namely the breast, to the hormones present in each woman's system.

An inadequate level of testosterone present in the young may lead to psychological inadequacy and a Caspar Milquetoast-type male. However, it must be pointed out and emphasized that deviation of sexual patterns, such as homosexuality, is not related specifically to abnormal hormonal levels. Indeed, many homosexuals, men in particular, are unusually well-developed males with adequate male hormone levels. The homosexual pattern is not governed by an adverse ratio of testosterone to estrogen. It would appear that the psychological aberration of the individual is responsible primarily for the sexual pattern that he follows. Of course, one knows that there is an ambivalence in all of us as far as sexual patterns are concerned, and in some this may result in "AC-DC" reaction by the male who may have homosexual propensities and heterosexual tendencies at the same time. This may occur in an individual who has a relatively unvarying testosterone level throughout his life.

In the adolescent adequate maturation of the genitalia, when deficient, may be readily achieved by the use of appropriate pituitary gonadotrophic hormones. These hormones may be produced from the pituitary gland, or, more commonly, from the urine of pregnant women. They have been most helpful in correcting testicular deficiencies which, if not treated properly and early enough, may eventually result in a nonresponsive male as the individual grows older. Once full growth is achieved in a normal individual, it is very unlikely that further penile growth will be obtained by intense hormone therapy. After the patient has reached his full somatic growth, then the hormone of choice, if there is a deficiency, probably would be testosterone per se.

Wise use of testosterone in individuals in the middle and elderly age groups who are deficient in male hormones has resulted in transformation of the individual from an inadequate, self-effacing, nonassertive, retiring individual to a very dominant one. The capacity for work is increased both mentally and physically. Interaction with one's peers becomes less abrasive and more tolerant in the hypogonadal male who has been given replacement therapy with testosterone.

The infertile male is still an enigma as far as therapy is concerned. True, while most progress regarding infertility has been made with the female, there is evidence now that the use of human menopausal gonadotrophin may be helpful in enhancing spermatogenesis in the male with a deficient sperm count. Testosterone itself may have an ambivalent effect and may enhance sperm production in the male in whom there is a testosterone deficiency.

One may categorically say that man is a product of his hormone production. When the hormone levels are normal, there are usually no significant consequences. Nevertheless, adverse psychological effects may influence the response of the individual to his own hormones, as well as affect his testosterone production. When hormone levels are low, as proven by laboratory procedures, replacement with appropriate hormone therapy may change the individual from an antisocial, unhappy person to a very agreeable, socialized individual who is well accepted by society and his peers; from one incapable of conjugal relationships to one who may be a satisfactory sex partner.

Two bugaboos continue to exist in the minds of many laymen and some physicians regarding testosterone therapy: the risk of cancer and the atrophy of the patient's own testicles upon continued hormone administration. To some extent these two questions have been responsible for the decreased use of testosterone in medical practice, following a period of great enthusiasm for the hormone in the 1940s. But in recent years there has been a marked resurgence of interest in the clinical use of the male and gonadotrophic hormones in the sexually deficient man, and that undoubtedly reflects a more knowledgeable and sophisticated approach to hormone therapy.

As we are now learning, with regard to the female hormone, estrogen, and its indicated relationship in some cases to cancer, inappropriate administration of any agents as potent as hormones can sometimes result in disaster. The final story in the female has yet to be told. Suffice it to say that the use of estrogens in the female with adequate safeguards, including the use of progestins, can alter the endocrine status of the female to create a much happier, physiologically normal individual without exhibiting an increase in cancer of the female reproductive tract. The same can be said of testosterone: There is no evidence that the hormone causes cancer. In fact, unlike the female hormones, testosterone has not been linked to *development* of cancer, although there is contradictory evidence that it may enhance the growth of cancer already existing in the prostate.

Concerning testicular atrophy, it is true that continued administration of testosterone will cause the testes to reduce or cease their own hormone production. Usually when treatment is discontinued, testicular hormone production resumes, often reaching levels higher than those before treatment. That is known as the rebound response. Yet, on occasion, testicular function does not rebound.

To stress that fact, however, is to beat a dead horse. Unless a deficiency of the hormone exists in the first place, a man should not be treated with testosterone for a prolonged period. If there is a deficiency, and if testosterone is the treatment of choice, the testes are already functioning inadequately.

Mr. Bahr has presented such facts as these succinctly and in a most readable manner. His book is to be commended, for it has separated fact from fiction and gives the reader a clue as to how effective his physician can be in correcting serious underlying endocrine glandular deficiency in the male.

New York City, HERBERT KUPPERMAN, MD, PhD

1
Do You Need Some?

At least a hundred thousand men in the United States are at this moment maintaining their masculinity with the help of a chemical. You could not guess who they are, and they probably wouldn't tell you. But they are scattered across the country in every large community. The hairy-chested mechanic who repairs your car could be one of them. The balding police officer, the young physical education teacher just out of college, the preacher, the local tycoon—all may have one thing in common.

For one reason or another, their bodies fail to maintain a sufficient amount of the male sex hormone, testosterone. The symptoms may be relatively minor—accumulation of fat around the breasts, inability to build muscle and shed baby fat, a higher than normal voice, sparse body hair, some fatigue and lassitude. Others have lost all interest in sex, and perhaps the capacity for it.

An estimated 10 to 30 percent of the men in this country are plagued with so-called potency problems on a more or less continuing basis. That, too, is sometimes caused by testosterone deficiency.

The greater the deficiency, the more pronounced and serious the symptoms: significantly underdeveloped penis and testes; a clearly feminine physique and voice; complete absence of body hair, except perhaps in the pubic area and underarms; and gynecomastia, or abnormal breast development.

Such extreme deficiency signs are easy to recognize, but much more common are the subtle indications of chronic low-level testosterone deficiency—irritability, indecisiveness, passivity, anxiety, fatigue. We all know the middle-aged man who suddenly could no longer cope, whose depression and anger and confusion destroyed his career, and perhaps his marriage, at that prime age in his life when both should have been richly fruitful. Ask him about it and he will tell you, "I don't understand it. I guess I'm crazy. I'm just not myself." And he's right. Hormonally, he's different from the man he was.

In the absence of any dependable studies, at least one authority estimates as many as eight to twelve million men in this country suffer one or more symptoms of insufficient testosterone. For the fortunate hundred thousand who are now receiving testosterone supplements, the results are often dramatic.

One such man lives in an obscure village deep in the Pocono Mountains of northeastern Pennsylvania. Lately he has become the talk of the villagers, and during the summer, when the vacationers arrive, they, too, sometimes hear about him. Reds is an ordinary man, good-looking with reddish-brown hair and clear brown eyes. His body is muscular, as well-developed as an amateur weight lifter's, although he has never lifted weights in his life.

Two dogs and a cat share the bungalow with him half a block from the main street of town. He owns five acres there, but most of it is in timber. The trees surrounding the cottage give him privacy. The barn, garden, and chicken coop all snuggle securely next to the cottage in the half-acre clearing, and that's sufficient.

Twelve years ago Reds' wife died. For half a decade he mourned her, became a recluse, and would not even walk the half block to the center of town for a haircut or a glass of beer. One afternoon a friend came to visit. Reds was dying of malnutrition.

The local doctor, a veteran of thirty years' practice in the county, found his patient hollow-eyed and pallid. The skin sagged from his bones. Reds spoke in dull monotones.

The doctor suggested hospitalization. Reds refused. Without a word, the doctor turned and left. An hour later he returned with a half dozen bottles.

"These are vitamins and minerals," said the physician sternly. "I want you to take five of them a day. And I want you to eat as much red meat as you can pack into that stomach of yours. And these . . ." He held up a bottle of small red tablets. "These are to help your appetite. One a day, every day."

He stared at his patient with calculated meanness: "Now you *do* it, or so help me I'm going to put you in the hospital!"

Reds listlessly began following the doctor's instructions. Within a few days his attitude improved. His appetite increased enormously. He walked to town every day to buy meat, and finally bought a steer and butchered it. He decided to paint the cottage and then build a chicken coop. He landscaped his half acre. Within three months he had gained back all the weight he had lost, but now it was chiseled muscle tissue, not loose, flabby fat. Then, for the first time in the years since his wife had died, Reds began to crave a woman. Today he sees one regularly. He has the time. He is seventy-three years old and has been retired for eleven years.

In mind and body Reds is thirty years younger than his chronological age. Everyone who knows him agrees that it is a miracle, a chemical miracle performed by a genie as unassuming as a bottle of small red pills—testosterone, the male sex hormone. Perhaps no drug has been more maligned, or praised, than testosterone. It stands alone today as probably the only true aphrodisiac in existence, and thousands of men like Reds owe their vigor and potency to it.

A twenty-six-year-old New York City accountant is typical of many thousands. One evening, after an exhaustive day at work, he met a woman in a Manhattan bar and picked her up—or rather, she picked him up. He had already decided against inviting her to his apartment when she asked him to hers. She was older than he by at least a decade. He disliked her perfume and the thick makeup she used to hide the wrinkles. Even her bright red lipstick annoyed him. But opportunities don't come that often, and what's more, he thought it would be unmanly to refuse. So he went.

Nothing happened, literally and tragically. He watched her undress and, unexplainably, he felt no erotic stimulation whatsoever. He stripped off his clothes, they climbed into bed, she fondled him, and orally teased his genitals. Yet he could not produce an erection.

Suddenly he was overwhelmed with shame—the height of the "unmanly." He dressed and left immediately, apologizing, claiming an upset stomach.

For more than a year that one experience totally destroyed the accountant's sex life. Each time he dated a girl, the thought obsessed him that he would fail if he tried to have sex. And, of course, by conditioning himself to believe that, he guaranteed failure. Finally, desperately, he visited a well-known New York City endocrinologist and sex therapist. The doctor discussed with him the causes of his original failure and helped him to understand that the aversion to that particular woman, no chronic failure on his part, had caused the original problem. Then the physician prescribed testosterone, one heavy dose the day before his next date.

The following night he had planned a gala evening—dinner, a movie, dancing and drinking, and then his apartment. Fortunately the girl, one he had dated regularly for several months, agreed to settle for the dinner and the apartment. There, a momentary fear, a resurgence of lust, and the potency problem was permanently abolished.

For more than a decade now women have been increasing their femininity, and in some cases actually reversing the symptoms of aging with female sex hormone supplements. By giving women the quantity of estrogen that the body, if it were functioning normally, would produce itself, practitioners such as Robert Wilson, MD, have eliminated menstrual cramps, regulated menstrual cycles, and restored physical vigor and happier outlooks. Yet, although books and magazine articles on female sex hormones have saturated the reading public, the average man remains completely uninformed concerning the degree to which the male sex hormone, testosterone, can help him attain, maintain, or reclaim his masculinity, youth, and sexual prowess.

Today, after eighty years of campaigns by fanatically zealous advocates and equally devoted detractors, the male sex hormone is beginning to receive the scientific attention it deserves. In hundreds of research facilities here and around the world, investigators are learning answers to questions thousands of years old: How do the testicles promote lust and sex drive? Why is a woman less strong than a man? Why are their sex drives different? What makes a man aggressive? Why are some men muscular and others flabby or scrawny?

To a great extent endocrinologists, through their research on the male sex hormone, can answer those questions and hundreds more. For the first time we are beginning to understand from a biochemical viewpoint what manhood is all about and the central role testosterone plays in it.

For all its importance, testosterone is no panacea or miracle solution to all the problems of manhood.

—No, it will not cure all sexual impotence, probably not even the majority of cases. But it will dramatically abolish those caused by the hormone's deficiency.

—No, the male hormone will not routinely cure depression in men. But some men, when they reach a certain age, suffer depression related to testosterone deficiency. The hormone can help them.

—Yes, there are factors other than hormonal which cause effeminate behavior in men. Yet, although it rarely happens, effeminate men can become more masculine by using testosterone.

If testosterone is not a panacea, neither is it an innocuous entity of the cough drop or vitamin pill sort. The testosterone made in a laboratory is a drug, available legally only by prescription. It is potent and can have far-reaching and sometimes undesirable effects. For example, although testosterone absolutely does not cause cancer of the prostate, there is some evidence it may enhance the growth of a cancer which already exists. Only a trained physician, ideally an endocrinologist, can determine in individual cases the need for the hormone and the proper dosage.

Another reason qualified medical supervision is essential is that whenever a hormone drug is taken for an extended period, the body's capacity to produce that hormone naturally decreases.

Thus a man's own testes will produce less testosterone than otherwise if the man is receiving the hormone synthetically.

Ordinarily that would be no cause for concern, for a doctor would not be prescribing testosterone if the man's testes were functioning adequately in the first place. What's more, when testosterone supplementation is discontinued, a rebound response usually takes place. That means that the testes, after a period of relative inactivity, will once again begin producing normal amounts of the hormone. We will discuss this in more detail later.

Today's endocrinologists know, as researchers only a decade ago did not, the wide variation in testosterone levels in every man. They've learned its relationship to a man's appearance, the size and health of his sex organs, its interrelationship with his sex life, and the effects food, drugs, and exercise have on the hormone's production.

Often, even today, the findings are in conflict, paradoxical. Without exception the research is complex, a maze of blind alleys, obstacles, and detours.

Yet the maze is profoundly worth traversing, for its dim terrain is the very genesis of manhood and womanhood, much of the root of our sexuality, our psychology—or psychobiology. We are quite literally what our hormones have made us. That is true of our bodies, our personalities, our gender—our sexual identities. Although the environment can modify us, sometimes radically, we are basically the product of our biology, including our hormones.

And that's where we must begin—with our hormones, the endocrine system—if we are to understand the testosterone maze.

2

Where the Action Is

Think of it: twelve small clumps of tissue scattered throughout the body. The largest weighs less than three slices of bread; the smallest could fit on the head of a pin. They are called endocrine glands, and they help regulate virtually every function of your body.

The testicles are one of these glands. They are neither large nor small, as far as endocrine glands go, a pair of them weighing about an ounce. Unlike the others—the pituitary, the adrenal cortex, and such—the testicles are familiar to virtually everyone. Even a child has at least a vague awareness of the size, shape, and location of the testicles. They are the most public, the most visible.

The endocrine glands produce incredibly powerful secretions called hormones. The potency of hormones can hardly be exaggerated. A comparison: Only 3.5 millionths of an ounce of the psychedelic drug, LSD, an amount so small it is almost invisible to the eye, can send a man on a mind-blowing trip. Less than two pounds of the drug could do the same for the entire eight million residents of New York City. About forty pounds would turn on the whole nation. Lysergic acid diethylamide is among the most powerful chemicals known to man.

Yet some hormones administered in doses as large as 3.5

millionths of an ounce will cause such havoc with the human body that it could lead to death. Often, hormones produce dramatic effects in doses one hundred times smaller.

We are, in a very fundamental sense, the product of these awesome substances. Long before we are born, within days (perhaps moments) of conception, they begin giving the orders that put us together, dictating the strength and size of bone and muscle, and the makeup of our blood and brain tissue. Throughout life they control food utilization, body shape and size, digestion, and even the rate at which we breathe, perspire, urinate, and defecate.

Hormones govern the rate of our heartbeat. They help to mobilize our defenses against attack from heat, cold, bacteria, viruses, and incompetent bosses. If we stand by quietly while he raves, we are obeying the dictates of a hormone. If we tell him what to do with his job and walk out, slamming the door, we are also responding to a hormone.

Hormones help mold our personalities. In women hormones dictate ovulation, the days when conception can occur, the beginning of menstruation, and the degree of sexual desire.

Endocrinology, the science of hormones, is still less than a century old. In fact, it was not until the 1940s and 1950s that researchers made their most significant discoveries. Today endocrinology is a fast-moving and exciting science. With every new finding comes another host of unanswered questions, but what has already been learned has been immeasurably profitable:

—Hundreds of thousands of diabetics live, and live longer, because of insulin.

—Certain hormone-related developmental defects such as dwarfism and infertility can be corrected.

—In the past a diagnosis of Addison's disease was a death sentence. Today its victims can live relatively normal lives.

—Menopausal women need no longer suffer intolerable menopausal depression. Today they are finding renewed youthfulness and vigor.

—Today's knowledge of hormones offers hope for the aging man struggling against impotence, the young man with the same problem, the weak, the flabby, the effeminate—the list goes on and on.

Compared to other sciences, endocrinology has reached its breakthroughs in a rather slow, plodding way. And no wonder, for tracing the circuitous life history of a hormone is no simple task. In fact, in some cases it is impossible. No one is even quite sure how many hormones there are—probably about fifty. One gland alone, the adrenal, produces at least five.

There are nine known groupings of endocrine glands, and probably others not yet discovered. The known ones include:

- Three in the brain—pineal, pituitary, and hypothalamus
- Three in the throat—thyroid, parathyroids, and thymus
- Two in the abdomen—suprarenal (adrenal) and pancreas
- The gonads are the final set of endocrine glands

In women they are called ovaries and are located approximately two inches below the navel, one toward the left side and one toward the right. In men the gonads are called testicles or testes. One is a testis.

With all these glands secreting what amounts to liquid dynamite, the theoretical potential for disaster is obviously high. But disaster rarely occurs because hormone secretion is regulated by complex checks and balances. The pituitary gland, once called the master gland, plays a large part in this regulation. Roughly the size and shape of a jelly bean, the pituitary is located deep inside the brain, in the most primitive and little understood area. It is approximately level with the bridge of the nose, in the center of the head. Surrounding and protecting it on three sides, thus indicating its importance, is a casing of bone. Above it is the hypothalamus, a mysterious part of the brain with crucial responsibilities in the endocrine system. We will discuss it later.

The pituitary is a kind of foreman for the endocrine system. It passes instructions on to the other endocrine glands. To the thyroid, for example, it sends thyroid-stimulating hormone. That prompts the thyroid to secrete thyroxine, which is necessary for growth, development, and normal body metabolism.

A little too much of this hormone and the victim's metabolism speeds up; he loses weight, grows nervous and irritable. Too little and everything slows down; he gets fat and stupid, sluggish and lazy. If he is an adolescent, his growth may be retarded. Another thyroid hormone, thyrocalcitonin, influences blood calcium levels.

The parathyroids also help to control calcium, as well as another mineral, phosphorus. They do this through the hormone, parathormone, and it is so essential that a total deficiency will lead to a low level of calcium in the blood that will cause death in a few days through respiratory and cardiac failure.

To the breasts and ovaries of women who have given birth, the pituitary sends prolactin, and that stimulates milk production. Another pituitary hormone, somatotrophic or growth hormone, stimulates bone and muscle cells and, along with other essential substances, promotes growth.

Situated above the kidneys are the two adrenal glands, each about two inches long, one inch wide, and an eighth of an inch thick. They are surrounded by an enormous number of blood vessels, far more than most glands. Through those vessels, the pituitary sends a hormone—adrenocorticotrophin, or ACTH—to stimulate the adrenals. On signal from this hormone, the adrenals produce their own group of hormones, among them cortisol, corticosterone, the catecholamines, and certain male sex hormones—seventeen ketosteroid precursors and aldosterone.

Another word for male sex hormones, incidentally, is "androgens." *Andro-* is a Greek prefix meaning man, and *-gen* denotes genesis or generation; an androgen is a hormone that creates the characteristics of manhood.

As androgens go, those from the adrenals are weak; the most powerful of them is only about one sixtieth as potent as the major testicular androgen, testosterone. For the most part, when researchers use the general term "androgen," they are referring to testosterone.

The adrenals of women, too, produce these weak androgens,

which are essential to the female's development. Both male and female adrenals also produce very small amounts of estrogens, a group of hormones which promote female growth and development and are crucial to a woman's fertility and normal menstrual cycles.

We could all live without the contribution the adrenals make to our androgen and estrogen levels, but other adrenal hormones are more essential. One was discovered by British scientists in the 1890s. After pulverizing some animal adrenals, they injected the extract into a laboratory dog. Almost instantly the animal's blood pressure was pressed higher. For that reason the investigators called the elusive hormone "pressor substance."

Today the synthetic version is known as adrenaline. It is, in a sense, the ultimate pep pill. In an emergency it increases the rate of heartbeat and constricts the blood vessels so that needed oxygen and nutrients can be carried throughout the body much more rapidly. It causes a rise in blood sugar levels, providing energy so that muscles can work longer and harder. Adrenaline stimulates the brain to function more efficiently. Endurance increases.

Important as adrenaline is, two other adrenal hormone groups are even more basic to the body's survival. The most important of these is cortisol. It converts amino acids to the sugar we need for energy and helps maintain blood pressure. When our antibodies attack antigens, cortisol protects surrounding innocent bystander tissues from being damaged. And in the brain the hormones are apparently instrumental in maintaining alertness of thought processes.

The other essential adrenal hormone is aldosterone. In the days before scientists knew how to treat Addison's disease (adrenal failure), its victims could expect to live only six more months. Usually the precise cause of death was a combination of cortisol and aldosterone deficiency.

Aldosterone has one major responsibility—to retain salt in the body. If too much salt is lost, the body cannot retain water. The cells dehydrate. Blood volume, much of which is water, drops dramatically. Blood pressure plunges, causing death.

The thymus is a mysterious organ. Until recently no one was quite sure what it did or why it was in the body. Authorities were not even certain it was an endocrine gland. They had not discovered a hormone it secretes. It simply looked and acted like an endocrine gland. But recently it was discovered that the thymus produces thymosin. That hormone plays an important role in immunity—it is essential to the development of lymphocytes.

The pancreas is the largest endocrine gland, and it is well understood. Most of the organ secretes pancreatic juices into the small intestine, where they help digest fats, proteins, and carbohydrates. But scattered throughout the tissue that makes the digestive juices are little islands (islets), each formed by a clump of about one hundred cells different from the surrounding ones. Called the islets of Langerhans, they produce two hormones—insulin, which converts blood sugar to glycogen, which is stored in the liver; and glucagon, which forces glycogen from the liver and converts it back into the blood sugar which is essential for energy.

It is a lesson in cooperation of opposites that the Democrats and Republicans would do well to learn. But even in the little islets of Langerhans things do not always work out the way they should. Sometimes the insulin producers work too hard or the glucagon producers are lazy. Blood sugar drops. Hypoglycemia develops. In the extreme, the victim may suffer insulin shock, coma, and death. On the other hand, too much glucagon and/or insufficient insulin leads to the notorious sugar diabetes.

The pituitary, that tiny gland in the brain once thought the master gland of the body, sends two regulating hormones to another set of endocrine glands—the sex glands, or gonads. Without these two pituitary hormones the gonads cannot function. The first of the pituitary's gonad-stimulating (gonadotrophic) hormones is called follicle-stimulating hormone (FSH) because it stimulates the female gonads, the ovaries, to secrete estrogens. Later the estrogens cause the egg cell to develop in its little capsule or follicle.

But follicle-stimulating hormone is not just a female hormone. The pituitary glands of men also secrete it, and it has a very important function: it triggers the testes (the male gonads) to produce sperm.

The second pituitary gonad-stimulating hormone is called luteinizing hormone (LH). In women LH has a rather complex job. First, each month it stimulates ovulation and release of the egg. Then it prompts the ovaries to form another hormone, progesterone, which prepares the lining of the uterus to receive the egg which is traveling toward it. If sperm does not fertilize the egg, progesterone secretion ceases and the uterine lining dissolves, thus producing menstruation.

Just as the testes make use of follicle-stimulating hormone to produce sperm, they also need luteinizing hormone, for LH stimulates the interstitial cells of the testicles to produce testosterone, as well as small amounts of estrogen. (We will discuss this in more detail later.) In men LH is often called interstitial cell-stimulating hormone (ICSH) for obvious reasons, and that is the name we will be using hereafter.

In a lifetime the testes will produce only about four and a half ounces of testosterone; in a day seven milligrams—seven thousandths of a gram, or thirty-five thousandths of an ounce. Tissues other than the testes also produce testosterone—the liver, adrenal glands, prostate, and even the skeletal muscles. But the testosterone from all of those sources is less than five percent of that from the testes and is comparatively insignificant.

A mere four and a half ounces—yet, without it no man would exist, and obviously no woman.

3

One Man Down

All his life Dr. Charles Édouard Brown-Séquard was a tempestuous, eccentric genius. By 1838, when he was twenty-one, he had already determined to be a writer, had written a novel, and had set out from his home on the island of Mauritius to take the publishers of France by storm. Instead, he met a successful novelist who urged him to forget writing and study medicine. After a while Brown-Séquard took the advice.

It was not easy. His father had died before he was born. The boy and his mother had lived in virtual poverty on the money she earned as a seamstress. Yet, when he finally made the decision to study medicine, he undertook it with incredible zeal. His doctoral thesis, "Researches and Experiments on the Physiology of the Spinal Cord," earned him a permanent place in medical history because of the new information it revealed.

In the following decades he seemed driven by an insatiable hunger for change. He practiced medicine in America, fought a cholera epidemic in his native Mauritius, and became physician in chief of the National Hospital for the Paralyzed and Epileptic in London. He lectured in Paris, Scotland, Ireland, and the United States, and he served as professor of urology at Harvard. Back in Paris he edited a medical journal, then taught in Geneva, and then again in France. At the College of France he held one of the most prestigious professorships in the world.

So copious were his writings that a bibliography has never been compiled. His findings on epilepsy, like those on the spinal cord, are permanent contributions to the medical literature. When he was sixty-three, he received outstanding honors from Cambridge University.

But a fellow scientist who attended that ceremony wrote that Charles Édouard Brown-Séquard seemed to have aged greatly. Decade after decade he had plunged into new areas of research and new endeavors, traveling from country to country, absorbing new experiences like a glutton for life until his energy was all but spent. Thus his friends whispered, but Brown-Séquard apparently did not stop working. Instead, he plunged into a whole new area of study—glandular secretions. There was no science of endocrinology then. Hormones had not been identified and only a few of their functions were recognized. In fact, through one of his early experiments, Brown-Séquard himself proved that the adrenal glands were essential to survival.

Brown-Séquard's specific interest was the testicles and their secretion. He had good reason. He was more acutely aware than anyone that his body was aging and his health failing. His biographer wrote, "He was irritable, impotent, suffered from gastrointestinal troubles, and was plagued by urinary disturbances, and no longer cared to be surrounded by eager students from the laboratory." Yet he realized that in some way not yet understood the testes possessed an almost miraculous power to produce strength and virility and potency.

There was nothing new about that observation. No doubt even before recorded history man learned that he could abolish a young stallion's youthful fire and render him docile as an old man by castrating the animal. By the same method angry bulls soon bent their necks in submission to the yoke. For the same reason—to break the spirit—the castration of defeated enemies after battle was a time-honored bedouin tradition. Hebrews as well as Arabs practiced it, and the scriptures tell us that David brought back from war two hundred foreskins (variously interpreted as male genitalia) with which to purchase as a wife Saul's daughter, Michal.

The characteristic aggression and dominance of manhood were in some mysterious, perhaps magical, way associated with the testicles. Ancient man knew that.

He knew, too, that the physical characteristics of manhood—the musculature and strength, the distribution of body hair, the deep voice—somehow sprang from the testicles. It is said that in about A.D. 300 the Indian physician and author Susruta of India recommended that Hindus eat testicles to cure impotence. During the Middle Ages thousands of soprano boys were castrated to prevent their voices from changing. By the mid-eighteenth century about four thousand were subjected to the operation. Many helped comprise the papal choir of the Sistine Chapel.

Ancient man also knew that sex drive, fertility, and potency were related to the testicles. Making eunuchs out of slaves probably began in Asia as a simple means of protecting women from houseboys and slaves. The Romans carried the practice throughout Europe.

A least one religious sect, the Skopts of Russia, used castration and penectomy (amputation of the penis) to control sexual impulses, which they considered evil. The Skopts became prominent in Russia during the tenth and eleventh centuries, and by the eighteen hundreds one writer listed their number as 5,444. Of these, about 4,000 were men; and of these, 588 had both penis and testicles amputated. In 833 cases testicles alone had been removed. According to those who underwent the operation, sexual capacity, if not desire, promptly declined.

Charles Édouard Brown-Séquard knew about the many effects castration produced. He was almost certainly aware of the statement of Theophile de Bordeu, physician of Louis XV: "The testes give a male tonality to the organism . . . set a seal upon the animalism of the individual. . . . Not only each gland, but each organ of the body is a workshop of a specific substance of secretion which passes into the blood, and upon whose secretions the physiological integration of the body as a whole depends."

What's more, he may well have been familiar with an obscure report published more than forty years earlier in the *Archives of Anatomy, Physiology, and Medical Science* called, "Transplantation of Testicles." It described experiments done by Professor Arnold Adolf Berthold of Göttingen.

Considering the climate of the times, Berthold's experiments were rather courageous. Revolution was raging throughout the German states. There was a climate of change in the air. If students or colleagues had learned of his peculiar interest, he may well have been laughed out of the university. So he did his work secretly at night in his home.

The first step in his research was not in the least unusual. He castrated (caponized) four cockerels, a simple process followed by all chicken farmers to assure that the excess males will bear tender, juicy meat at market.

Following the operation, Berthold pinioned two of the cockerels to his kitchen table and incised their abdomens. Into each wound he carefully placed a single testicle, then closed the incision with sutures, and put the birds in separate chicken coops he had built in his backyard.

A week passed. Berthold studied the cocks carefully. There was no doubt the two ordinary capons were changing. They ignored the hens flocking around them. Their combs shrank and lost their bright red coloring. They grew fat and lazy. Yet the two with the testicle implants continued to behave with all the cockiness of young roosters. Each morning they woke Dr. Berthold with their deep-throated crowing, attacked other roosters, strutted, mounted the hens, and paraded their brilliant combs.

Thus far Berthold's findings were curious, perhaps even fascinating. Still, they proved nothing that had not been known already—that the testes maintain masculinity. But Berthold was not finished. He sacrificed his two "roosters" and reopened the old wounds. And the sight that he *failed* to see puzzled his scientific mind.

Berthold believed, as did all scientists of his day, that the function of all organs and glands is controlled by the mind through the nervous system. Yet he could not find the slightest evidence of nerve growth surrounding the testes. Somehow these glands had continued to promote masculinity in the castrated cocks, but not by the ordinary means.

What he did find, instead of nerve growth, was a great network of new blood capillaries between the birds' abdominal walls and the newly transplanted testicles. Later, when he sat down to write his professional report, he drew the logical conclusion: "The testes act upon the blood and the blood acts correspondingly upon the entire organism."

Thereafter, Berthold abandoned this particular research and his paper was ignored. But not, perhaps, by Brown-Séquard.

In 1869, some twenty years after Berthold's experiments, Brown-Séquard was already wrestling with the question of how a man whose testicles had lost the power to keep him virile and vigorous might regain that strength. Half in jest he suggested to an inner circle of scientist friends that perhaps injecting semen into an old man's blood might be the key. He was not serious about that, though, and never conducted experiments along those lines.

He did perform a series of testicular grafts on guinea pigs, however, attempting to rejuvenate older animals by implanting the testes of younger ones. The results were unimpressive. Then on June 1, 1889, he walked to the lecture platform of one of France's most prestigious scientific bodies, the Société de Biologie, and addressed his colleagues. Later, some of them were to recall that he seemed twenty years younger, his face was once more bronzed, and his eyes bright with feverish alertness. To his astounded audience he calmly explained that he had been injecting an extract of pulverized dogs' testicles into himself for some time and that the procedure had rejuvenated him.

"Everything that I have not been able to do for several years on account of my advanced age, I am, today, able to perform most admirably." He left no doubt that he was referring particularly to a return of sexual capacity. To appease the skeptics, he also took tests with a dynamometer and an ergograph. Both proved a surprising degree of strength and energy for a man of seventy-three.

The following month Brown-Séquard published his lecture in the *Archives of Physiology*, a medical journal which he edited. Then all hell broke loose. Scientists who had not met him since he undertook the treatments denounced him as a fraud, attributed his report to "senile, erotic imagination," and insisted the experiments were the obscene folly of a scientist in his dotage.

Partly through the publicity generated by the extravagant condemnation, news of Brown-Séquard's self-experiments circled the world. Journalists scurried to the old man's flat at 19 Rue Francois Premier in Paris. After interviewing him, they filed stories of his youthful fire, his vigor and sincerity. Headlines around the world shouted the news: "Fountain of Youth Discovered!" The wealthy aged of the earth converged on Paris to buy and beg Brown-Séquard's magic restorative.

They found a withered, discouraged old man slipping rapidly into senility. The great and original "Savant," as one biographer hailed him, had finally and utterly exhausted his powers.

Had he actually experienced rejuvenation? No, at least not by the method he described. For one thing the "rejuvenation" hormone is not *stored* in the testes, only manufactured there. Very little hormone could be extracted from pulverized testicles. What's more, the salt solution he used to extract the hormone from testicular tissues would have been ineffective. Today we know that. As the doubters insisted to his face, Brown-Séquard's month-long burst of youthful exuberance was entirely a placebo effect—he *believed* the injections would make him younger, and so, for a while, they did.

A few years later a dying Brown Séquard admitted he had probably fooled himself. But he had missed the truth by a hair's breadth. Today the accuracy of his claims is no longer important. What is significant is Brown-Séquard's attempt to replace the mysterious substances that those tired old glands, the testicles, once gave to the body. As a result, medical historians usually consider June 1, 1889, the date Brown-Séquard announced his rejuvenation, as the birth date of the science of endocrinology.

Yet it was not until the 1920s that the mysterious substance was identified. A shy, self-effacing organic chemist at the University of Chicago, Professor Fred C. Koch, was quite certain that in one way or another at least *some* of the chemical produced in the testicles and responsible for masculinity could be extracted and identified, given the right procedures. Koch was a peculiar human being in that he had not the slightest desire for the traditional fame and fortune. He was simply a professional who felt he had a problem in need of a solution, one that, because of his training, he was as likely as anyone to discover.

In 1926, with the help of a young medical student, Lemuel Clyde McGee, Koch set to work. He knew that the chemical for which he was searching constituted an infinitely small part of a testicle's bulk—a needle in a city block of haystacks. So, in an approach far different from that of previous researchers, Koch decided to work not with an individual bull's testicles, but with tons of them.

He and McGee cooked, extracted, dissolved, fractionated and distilled day and night for three years. They awoke to fumes of ether, benzene, alcohol, and acetone. They retired with the smells in their nostrils. Finally, they injected the extracts into castrated rats. The substances were so impure that they killed the animals. Once they came close with a weak substance that caused the combs of castrated roosters to show some new growth. But the benzene used in extracting the chemical caused severe abscesses.

They made another batch, this time removing the benzene. The process was incredibly involved. The researchers started with forty pounds of bull testicles, grinding them into a mash, then extracting all the juices from them with alcohol for five days. An extract from the extract followed, using benzene. They removed the benzene by distilling, and then treated what was left with acetone. The result: twenty milligrams—less than a hundred-thousandth of an ounce—of some sort of acetone-soluble material. It had taken three years, but Koch and McGee had done it. The substance, injected into another castrated rooster, promptly transformed the bird's dull, sagging comb into a bright, upstanding red one.

McGee, the assistant, wrote the paper, giving it the somewhat less than dramatic title, "The Effect of the Injection of a Lipoid Fraction of Bull Testicle in Capons." Understandably, the paper stirred little interest, and since Koch's funding for the study had expired, he would have been forced to discontinue his research had not another professional shared his interest. The man was T.F. Gallagher, and, like Koch, he suffered a passion to produce once and for all the male chemical free from all impurities. Together, they started where Koch had left off, with the acetone-soluble powder. From that point, as science writer Paul de Kruif describes it, "They purified it further with the solvent, hexane, then shook it with alcohol, then washed the alcohol layer five times with hexane, then reextracted this hexane stuff twice again with alcohol, then again washed each alcohol layer five times with hexane, and then proceeded to transfer the material, soluble in alcohol, to ether, and shook it with alkali until it dissolved, and then shook that solution five times again with ether, and then shook that ether solution repeatedly with water. Till you'd swear that, after such an appalling chemical shoving around, whatever chemical will-o'-the-wisp remained would have forgotten that it ever came from the gonad of a bull."

That chemical was far more potent than the first—one hundredth of a milligram (one three-millionth of an ounce) injected daily produced a bright red comb on a capon in just five days. In 1929 Gallagher and Koch made known their findings to the scientific world. But Koch, typically modest, insisted, "The product is as yet grossly impure. We should not yet give it a name; too little is known of its chemistry. The chemical name would give us a false sense of security as regards the purity of our product."

That paper *did* get attention. Researchers across the country begged Koch for samples of his substance, and he worked around-the-clock to fulfill the requests. One came from a professor, A. T. Kenyon, a physician. Kenyon had a patient, a twenty-six-year-old man who had not developed normal masculine traits. He shaved but once every two weeks, and then only the inconsequential hair growth above his upper lip. Occasionally, but very rarely, he felt sexual desire. He had never ejaculated. His voice was high, his body hair almost nonexistent. Even his bones had failed to develop as they should in a normal adult.

Kenyon asked Koch if he could obtain enough male substance to use on his patient, and Koch agreed. From half a ton of bull testicles Koch supplied enough substance for fifty-three daily injections. In that short a time a transformation worthy of the term "miracle" occurred. The boy became a man. His body grew strong and new muscle began developing. Body hair developed. But the most significant change was in his libido. He developed a craving for sex and, simultaneously, the capacity to reach orgasm and ejaculate. Two months later his masculinity was once more fading for lack of Koch's substance. Yet the chemical's value in helping men achieve and maintain normal masculinity had been finally demonstrated.

By now news of Koch's work was spreading around the world. In 1931, a German chemist, Adolph Butenandt, processed nearly four thousand gallons of urine to obtain a substance similar to Koch's. Yet it seemed to be much weaker. What Butenandt did not know at the time was that he had not found Koch's substance, but the waste product released when Koch's chemical was metabolized in the body. The Butenandt product had only a fraction of the potency of Koch's.

The great practical breakthrough occurred in Amsterdam in the summer of 1935. Chemists working under pharmacologist Ernst Laqueur extracted from bull testicles what Koch had been seeking for almost a decade, a completely pure hormone. For the first time in history Laqueur determined the precise molecular structure of the male factor, the enormously potent substance without which manhood could not possibly exist. It was a steroid, a cholesterollike compound related to alcohol, but crystalline. It was the testis steroid, and there was no great expenditure of creativity in naming it testosterone.

A few months later, in Zurich, Leopold Ruzicka created testosterone synthetically. He used cholesterol, a substance so common and essential to life that it is found in every cell of the living bodies of animals and humans. Chemically, cholesterol is similar to testosterone. In fact, the testes themselves use cholesterol to build testosterone. (An irony: That which threatens life in the bloodstream helps create it in the testes, for testosterone is essential to healthy sperm formation.)

Now Ruzicka could use cholesterol to create testosterone in his laboratory. Because of that discovery, synthetic testosterone is plentiful and inexpensive today. It is available throughout the world in three major forms—pills, liquid injections, and crystal or pellet implantation.

Tablets are the most convenient and probably the most widely prescribed form of testosterone administration. The major drawback is that at least one oral testosterone preparation, methyl testosterone, may damage the liver if taken for prolonged periods. Pills and tablets are also less effective in reaching the bloodstream than other methods.

Injections of testosterone in a liquid base get into the bloodstream quickly and completely. The only disadvantage is that injections must be repeated every two to four weeks. That can prove time-consuming and expensive.

Implantation has the advantage of requiring only one visit to the doctor's office approximately every six months. The physician makes a small incision in the buttocks under local anesthesia, then inserts in the wound a tiny pellet of testosterone. The wound is closed with a single suture and there is virtually no pain. Thereafter, the pellet gradually dissolves, releasing into the tissue and ultimately into the blood small amounts of testosterone on a continuing basis. The process continues until the pellet is completely dissolved, which takes about half a year. For most men this is probably the most convenient approach. The only disadvantage is that precise dosage cannot be controlled, since a pellet's rate of breakdown will vary in some degree from man to man.

Tablets, injections, implantations—they are all being used, sometimes with dramatic effects, throughout the world today. If only Charles Édouard Brown-Séquard—and his critics—could see us now!

4

The Making of a Man

"The white-hot sperm explodes into the throbbing vagina in a dozen mighty jets of jism." Thus details the porno book writer. But the fact is, explosions are precious and rare, the jets are usually trickles, vaginas seldom throb, and sperm, if they have had a good day, might be lukewarm, but never white-hot.

Glorious as the paperback literature paints it, the life of a spermatozoan may be among the least enviable on earth. Born through a complex process in the tubes (tubules) of the testes, the spermatids, as the infant sperm cells are called, spend several weeks merely nursing on surrounding cells and growing. Eventually they develop whiplike tails and reach about 1/500 of an inch in length.

Finally, they set out—a half billion spermatozoan brothers—on the great journey of their lives. We might more accurately say brothers and *sisters*, for only half of them are potential males. The microscopic sperm contain an intricate coding device called the chromosome, containing the thousands of hereditary units, the genes. Every normal sperm cell has twenty-three chromosomes. From these, and from another set of twenty-three provided by the female's egg, fate selects at random all characteristics of the new child. Of the combined forty-six chromosomes, two are sex chromosomes. To distinguish between the male and female sex chromosomes, scientists label them with an X or a Y. The normal female egg always contains one X, or female, chromosome. Not so the sperm. It, too, may contain an X, and that would normally guarantee a girl—an XX combination. If, however, the sperm carries a Y chromosome, the child will become a male, or an XY.

So the sperm brothers and sisters, grown-up now but still sluggish with adolescence, set out on the first and last journey of their lives.

They pass into the epididymis, a small convoluted tube encased in tough protective tissue. Stretched out to its full length, the epididymis is about twenty feet long. Yet, in its casing within the scrotum, doubling back on itself continually, its length is about an inch.

Slowly, sluggishly, for ten to fifteen days, the sperm struggle through the twenty feet, maturing as they go. Then they enter another tube, the vas deferens, which continues for an inch and a half and then swells to form an ampul, a waiting station for the sperm, pending the journey's continuation. After conception seventy days must pass for a spermatozoan to reach maturity.

When sexual stimulation occurs, the sperm finally get excited about the undertaking. They begin dashing around in somewhat of a frenzy. Their behavior may be influenced by excretions from another organ, the seminal vesicles, according to some authorities. They secrete into the ampuls a sugar-rich fluid, and in some way the sugar may energize the sperm.

The intercontinental departure approaches. The sperm passengers slip into the urethra, the passage through which they will leave the male body. Surrounding the urethra on all sides at that point is a gland approximately the size and shape of an unhusked walnut— the prostate. The urethra runs through its center. As sexual stimulation increases, the prostate grows firm. Suddenly, usually at the instant of orgasm, it begins a violent spasming.

The sperm are instantly deluged with a milky, sticky fluid produced in the prostate and squirted out of it by the contractions. In an instant the sperm are swept up and ejected into a dark, sometimes friendly, sometimes hostile environment.

And that is the end. Every healthy spermatozoan struggles for survival against overwhelming odds. They are like salmon swimming upstream to reproduce and die, obeying some grand obsession, ripping themselves apart on the sometimes rough shores, preyed upon by antibodies, struggling and dying of fatigue by the millions upon millions. But unlike the salmon, almost none will reach the breeding ground. None will fulfill themselves by reproducing. For all half a billion sperm cells, the journey has been a tragedy, the one purpose for their existence unfulfilled.

For all—except one. One in 500 million! It swims upstream against gravity and the current caused by the beating hairs of the female reproductive canal. The gumlike consistency of the seminal fluid decomposes into a liquid, thus increasing the sperm's swimming ability. The closer it gets to the egg, the better its chances, for it seems the egg secretes a substance which attracts the sperm and keeps it moving in the right direction. Thus none of the 500 million ever attacks cells other than the egg. Invariably many sperm fall upon the egg simultaneously. None of them would ever penetrate, except that the egg's outer shell suddenly weakens. Perhaps enzymes in the seminal fluid cause the breakdown. Suddenly one sperm cell breaks through into the egg's interior. Immediately the egg's outer coating begins to harden again. The unsuccessful sperm continue their futile attack. Within two to five days after entering the vagina they will die.

But that one sperm will live and undergo a metamorphosis explainable intellectually, yet fantastic beyond our comprehension. Merged with the egg, it will become a single cell, a zygote, that will then split and become two cells, which will split to become four, and on and on with such repetition that at birth it will have multiplied to countless billions of cells, and at adulthood that sperm and egg will have multiplied to a quadrillion of them.

From the very beginning, presuming the sperm carries a Y sex chromosome, the zygote's natural tendency to develop into a female will be overwhelmed by masculine influences. Almost immediately in embryonic development primitive testes begin growing; and at sixty days they are recognizable, although little more than a network of tubes with a scattering of cells in the spaces between them. (Those cells are called interstitial cells, meaning "within the spaces.") The interstitial cells, also called Leydig cells, rapidly multiply, soon composing one half to two thirds of the young testes' volume. Then, a mere eight or nine weeks after the sperm and egg have united, the interstitial cells begin performing the chemical miracle of manhood—they start producing testosterone.

By contrast, the embryo which is not being masculinized has not yet even begun to show signs of femaleness. In the words of Dorothy B. Villee, MD, of the Harvard Medical School's Department of Pediatrics, "Embryonic gonads during this period are distinguishable as male and not-male, rather than as male and female." By the time a male fetus has developed a complete testes cell organization, the ovaries of a female fetus are just beginning to show female characteristics. Unlike the testes, the ovaries do not produce hormones in the embryo. Femaleness simply unfolds in the basic primitive evolutionary cycle.

Once the interstitial cells begin secreting testosterone, construction of the male sexual apparatus gets underway in earnest. Authorities disagree on the role testosterone plays in building the internal genital ducts—the seminal vesicles, vas deferens, prostate gland, epididymis, and so forth. But most authorities feel that androgens (male sex hormones), including testosterone, along with other secretions, do indeed bring about development of the internal male sex apparatus. They cite experiments in which fetal rats and rabbits were partially castrated—one of the two tiny testicles was removed. On the side in which the testicle remained, normal male sex glands and ducts developed. On the other side the tissues were female. In another experiment a testis was implanted on one side of a female fetus. On that side male organs developed. Since no "duct-organizing substance" has ever been discovered, these researchers presume it is some form or combination of the androgens, including testosterone, which trigger development.

The androgens of the adrenal glands, the 17-ketosteroid

precursors, probably also contribute to masculinizing the developing embryo. Although adrenal androgens are weak, compared to testosterone, they function in small measure in the same way testosterone does.

In fact, the relationship between the adrenals and the testes is quite close. In the developing embryo they seem to evolve from basically the same tissues, the testes eventually migrating to their permanent location. And they both produce the same male sex hormones. The testes produce about one third of the body's 17-ketosteroids, while the adrenals produce the remaining two thirds. The testes' primary secretion is, of course, testosterone, but the adrenals of both men and women also produce small amounts of the hormone.

Testosterone is a very powerful hormone, so much so that in excess it can cause defective development at certain stages of embryonic or fetal growth. The problem the body faces in controlling testosterone is somewhat analogous to that of an electric utility company sending half a million volts across the country in high voltage lines. All that power is essential, but if it ever flowed unchecked one morning into the family toaster, that would be the end of the toaster, the family, the house, and probably the neighborhood.

Utility companies use transformers to step down electricity's power. The body does the same. The liver is one of testosterone's transformers, and it reduces some of the testosterone produced in the testes to 17-ketosteroids. In the embryo as well as the growing child, those weaker androgens may contribute subtly but significantly toward the making of a man.

If you were to examine an embryo during the first two months of its existence, you'd not be able to tell its sex, for there would be no noticeable difference. The outer sex organs consist of a small nodule and, beneath it, a groove. On each side of the groove is a lump of flesh. If no testes are present to provide the essential hormones, the nodule will eventually develop into a clitoris. The groove will widen and split open to form the urethra and vagina with its inner lips. The surrounding mounds of tissue form the labium majorus, the large outer skin fold.

The testes develop as a kind of genetic mutation of the norm, and the androgens they secrete produce a radical transformation. The tiny nodule grows into a glans, the head of a potential penis. The groove fuses shut, forming a hollow tube, the urethra. Around it the mounds of tissue gather to produce the shaft of a penis. The bottom of the mounds enlarge to form a scrotum. For several months the testicles very slowly migrate toward the sac until, normally just before birth or shortly thereafter, they slip permanently into place.

Manufacturing a man is a very delicate process. Not only must testosterone and other androgens be present in particular amounts, but, even more important, they must be available at precisely the right time—in the early weeks of embryonic life. If the timing is off, even large doses of testosterone will not masculinize a fetus. For example, a twelve-week-old female embryo has already begun to develop a vagina. Then, no matter how heavy the androgen doses, the female anatomy cannot be transformed into that of a normal male. (Sometimes, however, the clitoris does enlarge—hypertrophy, as the doctors like to say.)

If testosterone is not available in sufficient amounts at the crucial time, many problems can result. One was well-known even to the ancient Greeks. According to myth, a son of the gods Hermes and Aphrodite went bathing one day and became permanently united in one body with a nymph. His name was Hermaphroditus, and today we describe a person possessing the complete genitalia of both sexes as a true hermaphrodite. The hermaphrodite has excited an enormous amount of interest and has been immortalized in literature, painting, and sculpture. Some of the sculptures are great works of art and are owned by the world's most prestigious museums. Two are on display at the Louvre in Paris; other hermaphrodites are at the Staatliche Museum in Berlin; the Museo e Galleria Borghese in Rome; the National Museum in Athens; the National Museum of Stockholm; the Barrow Museum in Rome; and the British Museum in London.

Without doubt, fewer hermaphrodites exist today than do paintings and statues of them. Less than a hundred authentic examples have been reported in the medical literature. And, historically, those rare people did not continue to exist long once their fellows discovered their dual sexuality because they were considered bad omens. The Athenians threw them into the sea; the Romans into the Tiber. Wherever they were found, they were put to death.

Among the more famous hermaphrodite legends is that of Catherine, or Charles, Hoffman, born in 1824, who was considered a female until the age of forty. According to a privately printed book, *The Hermaphrodite*, published for subscribers by the Erotica Biblion Society in 1903, Catherine, while still in puberty, had the instincts of a woman and lived with a man for twenty years. Her breasts were well-formed and she menstruated at nineteen. At age forty-six her sexual desires changed and she attempted intercourse as a man. That was so successful that she married and lived happily ever after. The story may be apocryphal, but it does emphasize the dual nature of the hermaphrodite.

Another story, this one very doubtful, involves a man arrested for prostitution. He was twenty-eight years old, five feet nine inches tall, and possessed well-developed male and female genitalia. He told authorities that he had given birth to a normal child. According to *The Hermaphrodite*, "In place of a clitoris she had a penis which, in erection, measured five and a quarter inches long and three and five-eighths inches in circumference. The scrotum contained two testicles, each about an inch long. She claimed functional ability with both sets of genitals and said she experienced equal sexual gratification with either. Semen issued from the penis, and every three weeks she had scanty menstruation, which lasted two days."

While the true hermaphrodite is extremely rare, pseudohermaphrodites are not. They are classified as male or female, depending upon which set of gonads they possess (ovaries or testes). Pseudohermaphrodites may appear completely normal. A female may have all the external characteristics of a normal woman. Only through internal examination will a doctor discover that she possesses no uterus or ovaries, only testicles producing a small amount of testosterone.

The reverse is equally common, the pseudohermaphrodite appearing to be a man but possessing the internal sex organs of a woman only—ovaries, ovarian ducts, and such. Often, upon close examination, the penis is found to be an enlarged clitoris. The usual cause of this is excessive production of testosterone during fetal life by the adrenal gland, and not testicular secretions. The biochemical and anatomic defects can be corrected and the girl can develop into a normal fertile woman. Slightly more of the hormone may permit penile development, but the urethral opening at the tip of the penis may instead be located at tne underpart of the shaft, a slight remnant of the vaginal opening which usually closes in the fetus under testosterone's influence. This problem, called hypospadias, is not at all rare. Usually the opening is only slightly lower than normal on the underside of the glans. Occasionally, however, the opening extends from the base of the penis to the scrotum, or, rarely, between the scrotum and anus.

Of great importance is the fact that both male and female pseudohermaphroditism, along with these other abnormalities, result primarily from insufficient androgen influence in the young embryo. Androgen deficiency, flawed timing of hormone release, and other as yet unidentified influences, can result in enough masculinizing hormone to produce internal male sex organs but not external, or vice versa. *Abnormal sexual development always results from a falling short in the progression from basic femaleness to masculinity.*

During the weeks following conception, androgen levels in male embryos vary greatly. John A. Resko of the Oregon Regional Primate Research Center in Beaverton, Oregon, has investigated androgen level variation in unborn male monkeys and has found that some have very low quantities in their circulatory systems, while others may have six times as much male hormone. Resko hypothesizes that some male fetuses are exposed to significantly more androgen than others, and that this variation causes a corresponding variation in degree of masculinity.

The difference is not all-or-nothing, but a degree of psychobiological sexual development on a sliding scale of masculinity.

Evidence from man's earliest existence shows that he has always recognized that not all men are created equally masculine. Yet only very recently has there been recognition—and scientific evidence to support it—that the same process which determines physical sexuality also produces psychic sexuality. And, just as there is a sliding scale of physical masculinity, so is there a panorama of sexual orientation among men, ranging from the exclusively homosexual to the utterly heterosexual. As with most research on the brain and its functions, evidence for sexual development in the fetal brain must come from animals. Yet there is good reason to suspect that findings with lower primates explain psychosexual differences in humans, too. We will discuss the studies and their implications later.

No one is sure why one male fetus may have a high testosterone level and another a low one. One safe guess is that testosterone production levels, like all other physical characteristics, are genetically programmed, the male embryo acquiring its testosterone-producing capacity from the genes of fathers, grandfathers, and great-grandfathers through the eons of its ancestry. Yet other factors—environmental ones—may play an equally important part, at least in some cases. For example, it has been determined that subjecting a pregnant animal to stress can cause feminization of the male offspring. On the other hand, a tumor of the mother's ovary may cause such excessive androgen secretion that a female fetus might be born with masculine characteristics such as a penis and an empty scrotum.

But these are insufficient explanations for the great variation in physical and psychological masculinity among men. Perhaps subtle factors in the mother's diet, her friendships, her attitudes, the climate, the time of year, and the sex life all affect the sea of chemicals, including hormones, which bathe the life in her womb throughout the nine months she carries it.

Whatever the cause of androgen variations, testosterone-dependent characteristics are set permanently in the early months following conception. And once the critical period has passed, even great quantities of the hormone will be ineffective in changing primary sex characteristics. An embryo deprived of testosterone, for example, will become female. If, during the fourth month of gestation, even large amounts of testosterone are administered, the infant will be a masculinized female, but always a female. The reverse is also true; no matter how serious the deprivation of testosterone after the first few months, a once androgenized fetus will always be male.

To summarize, nature's man-making process is anything but clear-cut and simple. It might be compared to our own striving for an ideal. Ideals are marvelous things to strive toward, but virtually impossible to attain—and that may be just as well for the world if we are to draw a lesson from the lives of those who have fanatically pursued perfection. "Pure" manhood, a human totally dominated by his androgen levels to the exclusion of all estrogen influence, has probably never lived. If he had, he would certainly have been a murderous, muscle-bound, bald, apelike boor too undisciplined to hold a job and, fortunately, short-lived enough not to care.

5
Half an Ounce of Manliness

For the nine months of fetal life nature pushes a crash program in sexual identity. Then, when the infant is born, sexual development virtually ceases. The interstitial cells, producers of testosterone in the testes, completely disappear! The boy infant has only minimal androgen in his blood to urge him on toward manhood. The infant girl is without estrogen in helping her develop femininity. Except for the obvious difference in sexual apparatus, girls and boys are quite similar in appearance and body build in their early years. There is no great difference in their ability to run, lift, or climb. The boy has about five percent more muscle. He is about twelve percent stronger. But his body is as smooth, and his skin as silky and hairless, as a girl's. He is no taller, no shorter, and he has almost the same amount of body fat and bone density.

The old nursery rhyme has it that boys are made of lizards and snails and puppy dogs' tails, and girls are made of sugar and spice and everything nice. While this is not quite true physiologically, it has merit based on sound observation: There are indeed some significant, if not physical, differences between boys and girls—*behavioral* differences. That once simple observation has been challenged in recent years by both serious writers and propagandists. They have argued that there is no innate difference in the ways boys and girls behave. They contend that children are conditioned by society to behave according to certain patterns. According to the argument, girls prefer to play with dolls because they are taught to prefer that. Boys choose trucks and guns and hammers for the same reason.

There is no doubt that what researchers call societal conditioning plays a very important role in all human development, including psychological, and we will have more to say about that later. But while armchair philosophers continue to publicize their own versions of psychological unisex, the overwhelming majority of research scientists quietly continue to view such impassioned pronouncements as simplistic and naive.

For one thing, psycho-unisex assumes a dichotomy, or division, between body and mind. That concept is obsolete. In fact, precisely the opposite is true. Some of the most exciting breakthroughs in medical science in recent years can be attributed in part to recognition that the brain functions according to biological chemical principles in the same sense that the liver, kidneys, heart, and lungs do. Thus many researchers are exploring therapies for mental illness which attempt to reestablish the brain's homeostasis, or chemical balance. We have learned that arguments with the boss can lead to mental tension, which in turn can cause chemical secretions which irritate the stomach linings, and which may ultimately produce an ulcer. We know that one of the early signs of some cancers is chronic depression. We know that some people literally die of grief, others of fear. We are not mind and body; we are body organs above the neck and body organs below. We are toes, spleen, brain, gonads, anus—and they work together as a single body to make us, hopefully, a nonschizophrenic whole.

If males and females are different genitally (and that, at least, has not yet been seriously questioned), then perhaps there are differences in other organs of the body, and perhaps in the tissues that make up the organs, and perhaps even in the cells themselves. In fact, microscopic analysis shows that is true.

In the child those differences can be traced almost exclusively to the presence or absence of androgens in the embryo and fetus.

During those formative prenatal months, the entire male body, including the brain, is saturated continuously with testosterone. And that exposure creates a permanent "masculine" imprint upon the male personality.

This masculine imprint includes a natural tendency toward aggressiveness. Uncivilized though such behavior may be, the male animal in the wild will kill or be killed for food, for sex, or for the pleasure of battle. And civilized man will do the same for land, money, pride, or power. Females will fight to the death, too, of course, but they do not have a *propensity* in this direction. Because of the high levels of testosterone continuously saturating the entire male body, including his brain, males are programmed to respond aggressively.

The first experiments attempting to demonstrate that involved rats and mice. In 1966, two researchers, Seymour Levine, professor of psychiatry at the Stanford University School of Medicine, and Richard F. Mullins, Jr., a graduate student, reported giving a single dose of androgens to a newborn female rat. It completely changed her outlook on life. Instead of desiring sex only when she came into heat, and then passively submitting to the male, she became a very passionate rodent. She attacked other mice sexually, attempting to mount them as a male would. What's more, she seemed unaware that female mice by nature build nests and stay close to home. Instead, she spent as much time running about and exploring her environment as the males did. The experiment was repeated with many female mice, and they all behaved the same way under the influence of testosterone.

In another experiment, D. A. Edwards of the Department of Psychology at the University of California injected testosterone into a group of newborn female mice. Into a separate group he injected peanut oil, which may sound curious to someone who is not a scientific investigator. The purpose was to establish a control group, mice which had been subjected to the pain and fright of the injection but had not received the testosterone.

When both sets of mice reached adulthood, they were all given testosterone. Eventually they were placed in cages, two mice together, for ten minutes.

For male mice that is a "war" situation. They will almost always fight. Females almost never do so. Yet ninety percent of the females who had received testosterone shortly after birth attacked each other. In contrast, only one pair of the peanut oil mice fought. Edwards varied the testosterone doses. The aggressiveness of the fighting females varied proportionally—those on low doses fought less; those on high, more.

Some people question the validity of these rodent studies, pointing out that a man is not, after all, a rat or even a mouse. So researchers switched to monkeys and came up with virtually the same results. Investigators at the Oregon Regional Primate Research Center injected pregnant female monkeys with testosterone and found that the female offspring behaved entirely like the male, and not at all like females. They invented new games, threatened and bullied the other monkeys, and went out of their way to get involved in rough-and-tumble play.

The monkey is a good animal for studies like this for two reasons. First, his physiology—the way his body is composed and the way it works—is similar to man's. Second, he is not subject to societal conditioning, as humans are. Thus girl monkeys who prefer dolls to trucks would not do so because mama monkeys told them that is how girl monkeys behave. Behavioral patterns in monkeys, as in most animals, are largely biochemical.

Dr. Robert M. Rose of the Department of Psychiatry, Walter Reed Army Institute of Research in Washington, D.C., has done probably the most informative studies yet on the relationship between testosterone and behavior in monkeys. Dr. Rose put thirty-four monkeys, all adult males, into a kind of puritan monkey heaven. They had plenty of space—more than a third of an acre. They had their fill of food and water. The temperature was maintained at an ideal level. They lacked only sex—no females were available.

Dr. Rose's study lasted nine months. During virtually all of that time, the monkeys simply lived together, interacted with each other, and watched Dr. Rose and his colleagues. The investigators, in turn, watched the monkeys. Lord, did they watch them! The researchers saw about eight thousand examples of behavior acting-out during the second, third, and fourth months, transferred their findings to cards, and fed them into a computer. Then, in the seventh month, they caught each monkey and analyzed its blood for testosterone levels. Rose's findings: The more aggressive the animal and the higher its position in group dominance, the greater the concentration of testosterone in its blood.

From the beginning of the study, when the thirty-four monkeys were first released into the large room, one quickly became the most aggressive. He frequently attacked the other animals and, with one exception, became the most dominant monkey of the group. He also had the highest testosterone level.

Some of the monkeys were not particularly aggressive. Yet they had a kind of masculine mystique which commanded the respect and submission of the others. This capacity to dominate was also significantly related to testosterone levels. In typical formal jargon Dr. Rose summarized his findings: "An animal's plasma (blood) testosterone is related to its dominance rank and the frequency of aggressive behavior exhibited in a social group."

But the human male is no more a monkey than he is a rat, as some of the more militant ambassadors of psycho-unisex have, no doubt with some reluctance, pointed out. Yet research with humans agrees with the animal studies. Dr. Leo E. Kreuz of Walter Reed Army Medical Center's department of psychiatry in Washington, D.C., and Dr. Robert Rose found that, of twenty-one prisoners, the ten with histories of more violent and aggressive crimes in their teenage years had significantly higher testosterone levels than did the other eleven without such histories. Said the researchers, "testosterone may serve to stimulate increased activity, drive, or assertiveness, and in some individuals this may be utilized in antisocial, aggressive acts."

Another study, this one involving a group of ten young girls, showed the same link between testosterone and masculine personality traits. During pregnancy the mothers of each of these girls were given male sex hormones as a treatment to prevent spontaneous abortions. The researchers, both specialists in pediatrics and psychology, are the well-known doctors Anke

Ehrhardt of the State University of New York, and Johns Hopkins Professor John Money. Writing in the *Journal of Sex Research*, they report that nine of the ten girls preferred boys' toys to girls', were more active than most girls in outdoor athletic activities, and had little interest in feminine clothes, baby care, doll play, or housewife games. If, as some might argue, these are simply liberated girls, whatever that means, then they were liberated by abnormal exposure to the male sex hormone, testosterone.

Similar studies could be cited at great length, but the point has perhaps been already over labored. Boys and girls, as well as men and women, are as different psychologically as they are biologically, and both differences result from the presence or absence of hormones. In the child that hormone is testosterone.

But, to repeat, the young boy's testes produce little of any male sex hormone. The masculine nature is set while he is a developing embryo in his mother's womb, and for the first eight years of his life, more or less, he drifts along on the manhood programmed into every cell of his body, but he is not particularly masculine. Certainly to some extent society encourages him to play a masculine role. Parents, friends, television, toy makers, and school teachers all encourage him to behave as men in our society behave. But if he is hormonally normal, he will not need much encouragement. Psychologists have noted tendencies from infancy for boys to be boys and girls to be girls in the traditional behavioral sense.

If anything, society may actually curb a boy's natural tendency to be his hormonal self. As we have seen, one function of testosterone is to produce aggressiveness. Male monkeys placed together will be at war within minutes. Two stallions, bucks, bulls, or mountain goats will fight, sometimes to the death and often without provocation. In that particular sense, then, our society does not so much teach a boy to behave in a masculine way as it does condition him not to behave in a way that is natural—and destructive—to the male of other species. (Society is obviously not completely successful in its efforts to demasculinize, in this respect, the human male beast. Thus war, rape, murder, and other violent crimes continue to exist, the overwhelming majority of these acts being committed by men.)

People grow faster in the first decade of life than at any other time, and they do so without any assistance from sex hormones. The thyroid hormone supervises bone growth, brain development, and even protein utilization. Insulin is essential for building muscle from protein. Insulin also encourages the buildup of body fat, which partly explains the typical child's soft, smooth body. The ultimate director of the whole show at this period is growth hormone, produced in the pituitary and affecting all the glands, organs, and tissues of the body.

This process of childhood growth is an amazingly complex and utterly marvelous thing—as far as it goes. But it does not go far enough. The child's body is the framing and foundation of the man or woman. It is an essential but incomplete part, and it requires a great deal of additional material. The girl needs estrogens and the boy needs androgens, primarily testosterone. Without those hormones children remain essentially children in a biological sense, no matter how long they live.

The drama of maturation begins secretly. The child is none the wiser. In an intriguing and still mysterious portion of the brain, the hypothalamus, something unique and fascinating takes place. Even today the first stimulus is so shrouded in the great primitive secrets of the brain that scientists have not been able to explain it. But suddenly the hypothalamus begins to send messages to the pituitary, located directly beneath it, via a hormone. It is called, logically, gonadotrophin (gonad-growth) releasing hormone, or GRH.

When the hypothalamus gives the order, the pituitary hops to it and releases gonadotrophins (gonad growth hormones). There are two of them, which we have already discussed in Chapter 2. Follicle-stimulating hormone (FSH) finds its way to those endless tubes in the testicles, the seminiferous tubules, and soon spermatids (infant sperm) begin to proliferate. The second pituitary gonadotrophin bypasses the tubules and settles in the interstitial cells between them. For that reason the hormone is referred to as the interstitial cell-stimulating hormone (ICSH).

The boy does not know about interstitial cells, probably is unaware that he has testes, knows only that there is a tight little pouch beneath his penis, and that together they form the one part of his anatomy that must absolutely not be displayed before others. Yet, for all his disinterest, as he approaches the teenage years, the interstitial cells begin to assert themselves. At first slowly, then in greater and greater quantities, they begin pouring testosterone into the blood. At first they work only at night, during the boy's deep sleep. The hormone floods his body, his brain. It stimulates the boy to dream of sex. He has his first orgasm, utterly baffling, immensely pleasurable, probably without ejaculation, for the testicle tubules and the prostate are not yet mature enough to make their contributions.

The testosterone washes through him and he staggers in bewilderment. His voice begins to crack and squeaks utterly out of control (he does not know that testosterone is stimulating the vocal cords to grow thicker, utlimately giving him a deeper, more powerful-sounding voice). He is shorter than almost every girl in his class. His chest is concave, his abdomen convex, his muscles weak—even his mother is stronger than he is. He begins tripping over his own feet, embarrassed no end at his sudden inability to control a body he had learned to master years ago.

But very quickly now the miracle of manhood unfolds. Testosterone, taking over where the thyroid hormone left off, has hastened bone growth along the way to its final maturation. In another handful of years the boy's bones will be strong and sturdy, and testosterone will have been responsible. When growth finally stops, that, too, will be brought about by testosterone. In women estrogen has the same function.

Normally, as the boy grows further into his teenage years, he will notice a change in his body composition. So-called baby fat will slip away as testosterone replaces insulin as the major promoter of tissue growth. Unlike insulin, testosterone discourages fat buildup and promotes muscularity.

There are other changes in the maturing adolescent, less obvious but equally crucial to approaching manhood. Testosterone stimulates kidney growth, and the kidney in turn contributes to more red blood corpuscle production. Hair sprouts from nowhere—in his armpits, above his penis, on his scrotum. Some fuzz even appears above his upper lip. His growth rate increases by fifty percent.

The boy makes a secret discovery: his penis is enlarging, his scrotum growing fuller, the testes becoming sensitive in a way they had not been before. He does not know what an epididymis is, a vas deferens, a prostate, or a seminal vesicle. They are the machinery of manhood, the equipment for sperm manufacture, transport, and delivery. They are growing, too.

The normal boy is not going to take very well to being called a boy any longer for he has experienced a glorious revelation. He is capable of orgasm. He can shoot sperm. For virtually every boy there comes a conscious moment of relief with this knowledge that he is normal and will be a man after all.

The young man evolves a new personality to go with his new body. Physician, teacher, and writer Dr. Gustav Eckstein, in his book, *The Body Has a Head,* calls this youth with flowering manhood the swashbuckler:

> Into the town comes the swashbuckler, has something to sell. That is his role, or his illusion. Assault is his physiology.
>
> He is the owner of two testicles. Carries them outside in front of him, a unique idea that even the male mind never quite gets used to...
>
> The swashbuckler, when he entered the town, carried with him his secondary sex characteristics—angular look, visible muscularity, low voice, a mind that touches with maleness everything that body touches, and a confidence born of the knowledge that he is possessed of the talent to keep life alive by fertilizing an egg.

He is the cocky, arrogant rebel. He hates his parents. It is a new personality—he has not yet learned how to round off the edges, to handle the immense power flowing through him, the concentrated, continually teasing, distracting power in his groin. For a time it is anyone's guess, including his, whether he is slave or master of the testosterone that makes him a man. Testosterone makes sex much more urgent and continuing for him than estrogen does for women. The combination of testosterone and societal stimulants renders the young man literally obsessed with sex. In their book, *Man*, Richard J. Harrison and William Montagna wrote:

> Among the unique biological attributes of the human male animal are his almost perennial concern with sex and his never-ending search for sexual experiences. Man has shrouded sex in dogmas, taboos, rituals, symbols, religion, fantasies. He has both sanctified it and reduced it to vulgarity. He writes poems about love, erects giant monuments, paints acres of pictures, carves mountains of stone, wood, and metal, subjects himself to torment and even death, and goes to war. His attitudes toward sex span the gamut from total denial to total indulgence, from infernal to paradisiacal. Man's fervor for sexual experiences, real and fancied, is reflected in his literature, most of which recounts his joys and sorrows in love.

Nature has a goal through those years of development. She strives to carve out an ideal man, and testosterone is the blade she uses, but sparingly—not more than half an ounce throughout adolescence. And man is in all his essence the product of his hormones. Says Dr. B. Ionescu of the Institute of Endocrinology in Bucharest, "Indeed, the male pattern, with all its morphological function, compartmental and social complexities, is entirely the work of the endocrine testis, which partially determines even its own spermatogenetic function."

His body is testosterone's hallmark. Normally, in adulthood, he will have a body fat content of twelve percent. His female counterpart will have about twenty-nine percent. His muscle will be more dense, his bones significantly stronger to support added weight and stress. He will be thirty-three percent stronger.

But manhood is not so simply explained. If it were, every man would have a biological right to be the swaggering macho beast. That is a role no male psyche has ever been truly comfortable with. It has been played as a cultural norm and throughout vast periods of history—overbearing he-man ruggedness and dominance; brutality for its own sake. Yet it has never been more than role playing and is often discomforting, frequently accompanied by social, psychological, and sexual problems.

The reason: The machismo role is out of tune with male

biology. Man is not merely the product of the testosterone in his blood vessels. He produces in his testes not only androgens but also estrogens, the female hormones. They, too, have an influence—and an important one—in producing a normal male. Nature attempts to curb the sexual extremes. Both the pale, fainting female and the emotionally ice-cold, rock-hard male have limited survival potential, for the woman will collapse under pressure and the man will explode under it. In a figurative sense estrogen is the rubberizing agent in both the body and the personality. An excessive amount in a man or woman makes for a flubbery, blubbery creature, unattractive and incapable of seriously functioning. On the other hand, insufficient estrogen produces a brittle, glasslike body and mind incapable of flexibility. It withstands what it can, then cracks and shatters.

6

A Hormone with Enemies

The machismo myth notwithstanding, masculinity for modern man exists on a precarious foundation. Through a complex psychobiological linkup, both the quality and the quantity of stress continuously bombarding modern man is performing a chemical castration that in some cases is only minimally less thorough than the literal surgery would be.

There are three kinds of stress that prehistoric man never confronted. One is the stunning sense of responsibility for worldwide circumstances. Only in this century has every man, from ditchdigger to international corporation president, learned on a daily ongoing basis of assassinations in Spain, earthquakes in Peru, starvation in India, bloody revolutions in Portugal, economic chaos in Britain, airplane crashes anywhere and everywhere they occur. The overwhelming avalanche of tragedy and horror tumbling from a single issue of a single newspaper today would equal half a lifetime of grief a mere century ago.

It may be that, in order to maintain sanity, the wise solution is to cancel all subscriptions to news magazines and newspapers, avoid the six o'clock and eleven o'clock news like the plague, and live in a vacuum. Some people accomplish that quite successfully. Others continue to expose themselves to the news, shake their heads sadly, and simply refuse to get involved emotionally. That is understandable. It is sane.

But the androgen-stimulated man is under a *compulsion* to act and to react. It is truly not his choice—it is his nature. He is a body of programmed aggressiveness, as we have seen. He cannot read of a brutal crime, political crookedness, environmental dangers, energy shortages, economic woes, wars, deaths, or injustices without reacting. Perhaps he will talk to neighbors, form a group, a lynch mob, an army, murder the guilty, the innocent. Perhaps he will only make a speech or write a letter. He may do even less, simply think about what is wrong with the world, brood over it, develop an ulcer or heart disease, and kill himself.

But as long as he is secreting normal amounts of androgen, he will be stimulated to interact with every problem that troubles him in his house and in his world, whether or not he acts upon the stimulation.

For this past century, more or less, the ordinary man has encountered another enormous source of stress, and it has gained great momentum in recent years. He has been faced with questions of his own worth. Once secure in the assurance that he was made in the image of God, man today stumbles through life with no image whatsoever. He is born void of destiny, nurses a computer to pay his bills, tightens a bolt on an assembly line until a machine can be made that will do it cheaper. In the extreme he will show his individuality through an explosion of violence, his sexuality through rape, and his aggressiveness through murder or the acquisition of wealth. But for the most part he will be a nothing, even sexually, for he has finally come to accept himself not as a workingman but as a working*person*, a spokes*person*, a neuter human being.

Through a grotesque miracle of guilt men today, particularly younger ones, are chronically apologetic concerning their manhood. Aware of, and properly concerned with, the injustices men have historically inflicted upon women, they have denied not only excesses and abuses of masculinity, but masculinity itself. They have docilely fallen in step behind the myth of psychological unisex, denying any kinship to traditional masculinity. The homelife of modern man is a montage of disrespect and defeat, a war of words, a battle for which he is not particularly well-equipped. Such weapons, from an evolutionary perspective, are perfectly new to him, and by his own decision he has outlawed use of that which is most primitive and natural to him—his brawn.

If some men have surrendered their masculinity, others have gone to the other extreme. The machismo we discussed in the previous chapter is the outward display of exaggerated manliness. It comes from the Mexican word *macho*, or male. But the macho is no ordinary man. It is conceivable that if Tarzan lost Cheetah, his chimpanzee, to a crocodile, the man might shed tears of tender grief. No macho would be seen displaying such weakness. Superman would never kill someone simply to defend his honor. A macho would *talk* about doing it, at least, even for his friend's honor. With women his slogan is, "Love 'em and leave 'em." Among American heroes, probably only John Wayne and King Kong fulfill the true machismo image.

Trying to convince the world one is the resurrected Christ could hardly be more stressful. Men *do* feel great sorrow and grief. Crying *is* a normal reaction. Often violence is neither enjoyable nor conducive to good health. Sometimes even the macho finds himself sexually impotent. Swearing, smoking, and drinking cannot change that. The machismo is a myth no man can attain—or should want to. Yet the man who is trapped in such a definition of his own selfhood fails to recognize that. All he knows is that he personally falls short of his ideal, and the knowledge condemns him to stress and despair.

A third stress to civilized man is the guilt arising from sexual self-pleasure. Even today the sex manuals contain an inordinate imbalance of instructions to men on how to please women as compared to guidelines for the female. The male has been conditioned to consider himself a failure if he surrenders to his natural impulse to simply mount and be done with it. Certainly no woman should be expected to tolerate chronic use of her body as a container into which a man routinely masturbates. Yet anyone with a modicum of sexual experience need not rely on the psychology texts for evidence that there is a significant difference between sexual compulsions in men and women. The estrogenic female has a slower-developing, more thoroughly pervasive and longer-lasting erotic desire, the male an immediate, compulsive, and demanding one. Should today's man, in a moment of weakness, yield to his "bam, bam, thank you, ma'am" nature, he will likely experience both guilt and anxiety. Guilt because he has not only considered his own needs first, but exclusively, which proves him a male chauvinist pig. Anxiety because the *real* man (shades of the machismo) never fails to give his woman at least one orgasm, preferably a half dozen.

Thus the aura of sexuality has changed for modern man. Says psychiatrist Harvey E. Kaye, MD, "It has been the unhappy fate of the contemporary male and his well-intentioned phallus that his sexual center has been insidiously forced upward from the crotch toward the brain." Millions of exceptions notwithstanding, most men—and women—remain today, as they have historically, sexual victims of their conscience and their conditioning. Only the few can enjoy what Kaye calls recreational sex—"enjoyable play, happily hedonistic. . . . A phallic frolic, it is of no cosmic import, and free of compulsivity, imperatives, and guilt. It can be identified by adjectives such as 'lusty,' 'earthy,' 'lecherous,' 'sensual,' 'voluptuous,' and dozens of other intriguing terms which have unfortunately acquired a pejorative connotation in a togetherness-centered culture which is committed to the containment of recreational sex."

Instead of a phallic frolic, most men undertake a penile performance, often with disastrous consequences. It could hardly turn out otherwise, for, in efforts to stimulate his partner sufficiently, hold back his orgasm, and control his natural instinct to dominate, he is in effect suppressing the expression of his libido and his masculinity. Sex activity itself soon generates significant stress.

The startling irony is that all stress *reduces testosterone levels.* Thus nature maintains a natural psychobiological homeostasis, a harmonious stability. The man driven to great concern because of crime, crooked politics, world problems, or personal debt develops a decrease in precisely the hormones which trigger his unrest. He grows apathetic, dispassionate. The machismo grows less and less capable of playing his synthetic role. The man who finds sex stressful will likely experience a decreased sex drive.

To understand how emotional stress affects hormone secretion we must understand the *hypothalamic-pituitary-gonadal axis*, the roundabout method whereby testosterone secretion is stimulated. We know that the pituitary, the master endocrine gland, secretes gonadotrophins into the blood, and these stimulate interstitial cells to produce testosterone. But, as we have mentioned, the pituitary does not function according to any independent capriciousness, but obeys very faithfully the dictates of a section of the brain just above it—the hypothalamus.

If humans are anything more than biochemical robots, if somewhere within us the mechanistic interactions of nutrients, enzymes, and other chemicals fall under the control of the selves we *think* we are, that assertion of our "personhood" occurs in the hypothalamus. It is not even an independent organ; it is merely the basement portion of the midbrain, with no clearly defined boundaries and no outstanding visible features. It composes only three tenths of one percent of the brain weight. It has a long history, was a part of the human anatomy before there was such a thing, before what is now man could rationalize, speak, and think. Long before those more "modern" portions of the brain evolved, the hypothalamus was regulating the prehuman's most basic biological activities, his hunger, thirst, and libido, and was controlling his blood pressure, heart rate, body temperature, water balance. The hypothalamus was interpreting certain sensations as pleasurable, others as painful.

There is nothing particularly unique in that—many areas of the brain control very specific bodily functions. But the hypothalamus alone performed the awesome conversion of nervous impulses to chemical instructions.

You are walking alone in the woods. A cool breeze develops. The nerve endings in your skin send the message to your brain that you are cold and losing body heat. Ultimately nerves take that message to the hypothalamus, the major nerve terminal. Robert Williams, MD, author of the prestigious *Textbook of Endocrinology* used in many medical schools, calls it the "head ganglion," a gathering place for nerve cells, a center where nervous impulses are discharged. Receiving that information, the hypothalamus can respond in two ways: It can send out its own nervous impulses, stimulating the raising of body hair to control heat loss; or it can, *through chemical secretions*, increase blood circulation to maintain core body temperature.

Fear, anger, lust—all our conscious emotions apparently reach the hypothalamus. Says endocrinologist/author Robert Wilson, MD, "The gasp of horror, the breath held in suspense, the pupils enlarging in surprise, the flush of embarrassment, the sweat of anxiety, and the heart pounding in fear—all these are evidence of this (hypothalamic) mind-body link."

The hypothalamus is continuously busy sending messages, in chemical form and via the bloodstream, to the pituitary: "Tell the adrenal glands to secrete adrenalin! More thyrotrophin! Less aldosterone!"

Sometimes input from the conscious world via the nervous system is so excessive that the hypothalamus overworks. Says Wilson, "Nervous tension, by acting on the hypothalamus, can produce digestive disorders, including gastric and duodenal ulcers, diarrhea, and colitis. It may interfere with the functions of the liver, pancreas, and kidney, causing dangerous accumulations of toxic substances in the body. Bladder functions can be similarly affected by emotional disorders."

Thus, for both better and worse, emotions can affect hormone secretions. Specifically, both physical and emotional stress trigger the hypothalamus to order the pituitary to cease stimulating the testes. And that brings about a decrease in testosterone levels. Researchers at the Walter Reed Army Medical Center in Washington, D.C., proved that some years ago through a study involving three groups of soldiers. One group was in basic training at Fort Dix, New Jersey; another was undergoing special hazardous conditioning in the mountains of Vietnam; the third group was living a relatively normal life. That third group had the highest testosterone production levels, followed closely by the men at Fort Dix. The Vietnam troops, who were in constant fear of attack and destruction, according to the researchers, produced significantly less testosterone than the others.

A follow-up study by Walter Reed investigators was published in May, 1972, in the *Archives of General Psychiatry*. This time the subjects were eighteen young men undergoing the Officer Candidate Course at the U.S. Army Infantry School in Fort Benning, Georgia. The emotional pressure the trainees faced was intense. It was planned that way. According to the *Infantry Officer Candidate Manual*, "The application of pressure is one of the key techniques in the leadership development of an officer candidate." So severe is the stress that in recent years about one in each three trainees has dropped out of the program before completion.

The studies were made when stress was at its highest, during the program's third week. Following routine tests to establish that the candidates were indeed feeling severe stress, their testosterone levels were examined. All but one were at least ten percent lower than could be expected in normal men. One was sixty percent lower. They averaged a decrease of about thirty percent. The investigators, under the leadership of Major Leo E. Kreuz, waited several weeks and then repeated the tests. At that time, as expected, the program had grown less intense, and the candidates more confident. In psychiatric interviews they reported, "The program is very relaxed. All the pressure is off," and similar attitudes. Their testosterone levels then had bounced back to normal, even surpassing those of ordinary Army volunteers used as controls.

Concluded Dr. Kreuz, "The results of these studies were clear: Plasma testosterone was significantly lower during the stress period. We believe that this represents the first evidence in humans suggesting that psychological stimuli suppress levels of circulating plasma testosterone. . . . The officer candidates were more outgoing and expressed higher levels of sexual interest and activity during the recovery period."

Long before the Walter Reed studies, researchers found conclusive proof in animals that emotional stress reduced testosterone production. In fact, stress in male mice actually decreases the weight of the testicles. Monkeys suffering stress produce much less testosterone than they otherwise would.

Stress not only reduces testosterone production, but also

permits the female hormone, estrogen, to take a more active role in the man's psychobiology. To repeat a point made earlier, the normal testicles produce not only testosterone but also minute amounts of estrogens. What's more, the male body actually converts small amounts of testosterone into estrogen. Just why is unknown, but recent studies suggest that estrogen may have a very important function in the complex hypothalamic-pituitary-gonadal axis.

Obviously, if the hypothalamus continued to signal the pituitary to signal the testes to produce testosterone, men would be overcome with the critically high levels of male hormone. For that reason scientists have realized for many years that a feedback system must exist—somehow the hypothalamus must receive a signal when blood testosterone levels are sufficiently high, and that causes it to stop sending orders to the pituitary. Preliminary findings indicate that it is not the testosterone alone which signals the hypothalamus, but also estrogens produced along with the testosterone.

But estrogens and androgens are competitors, each fighting for the same special proteins to carry them through the blood, each seeking the particular enzymes needed to convert them to more useful forms. In effect, estrogens and androgens carry on the eternal battle of the sexes, each trying to dominate the other.

Although stress causes the testosterone levels to decrease, estrogen secretions may continue unabated, and that can often lead to estrogen-related effeminacy. That point is much too significant to be dismissed in so cursory a way, and we will elaborate on it hereafter. But for now it is enough to say that estrogen, produced normally in a man's own body, is, when in excess, the enemy of his testosterone.

But it is a secondary enemy, adversely affecting masculinization only after other factors have reduced testosterone production in the first place. The primary enemy is *stress*, the stress of everyday living, the stress that pursues the victims of Toffler's *Future Shock*, and the American Heart Association's cardiac attack profile, and the Alcoholics Anonymous alcoholic profile. Stress is a far more serious threat to masculinity as we know it than any other sociological factor.

The man who finds effeminacy subtly encroaching upon his manhood may simply be suffering the effects of stress. Rather than allow that problem to add to his pressures, he would do well to analyze the sources of stress in his life and take steps to eliminate those that are not necessary to survival. One man sold a huge showcase home with outrageously expensive upkeep and high mortgage and bought a row home with the equity in his first property. Although he lived more simply after that, he began feeling like a rich man overnight, and knowing he was able to bank a couple hundred dollars a month relieved him of great stress. Another man quit a job he had held for twenty-two years and took another at one third less pay—and responsibility. Two years later he was still elated by his decision. For him it was a matter of survival, not only as a human, but as a man.

7
The Search for an Aphrodisiac

"I don't eat especially because I'm hungry; I know it is more than that. I have a lonely hunger. I eat sometimes because I don't have anything better to do. I am a very lonely person, and being in this room makes it much more so, and I am much more susceptible to eating."

The letter was written by a twenty-four-year-old man to an endocrinologist because he did not have the courage to discuss his problem face-to-face with the doctor. "Another thing that bothers me constantly," he wrote, "are the fat, flabby breasts. While walking around in a T-shirt they protrude, and I am embarrassed. I have never had intercourse and know I could never bring myself to do so. In fact, I can't even bring myself to ask a girl for a date. In other respects I have no fear of them. I talk and kid, but that is as far as I can go. In fact, I feel that I will never have the nerve to ask a girl for a date."

Harry L. discovered his own problem when he was fourteen. He noticed his body was not developing as it should. His genitals were smaller than normal, his body flabbier, and he had almost no pubic hair growth. When he was inducted into the Army, the examining physician told him he needed medical treatment, but he was embarrassed to see a doctor. During the entire two years he was in the service, he managed to keep other soldiers from seeing him naked, and so avoided being teased.

By then he had made up his mind to live the life that nature had apparently destined him for—one of isolation, with no close friends and absolutely no hope of an active sex life. That in itself caused him no great concern. He had never felt a strong sex urge. But one matter drove him practically to distraction—"I got tired of being treated like a young kid."

After he was discharged from the Army, Harry could have found any number of well-paying jobs for he had a Performance Scale IQ of 123—very superior. But he settled for a janitor-errand boy position in a local hospital. That is where he met the endocrinologist and, by letter, revealed the truth: He was not only physically immature, but totally impotent.

With respect to impotence Harry L. is not as alone as he imagined. Writes Harvey E. Kaye, MD, a New York City psychiatrist, in his book *Male Survival* (1974), "It appears that the male's emotional estrangement from the erotic is rapidly assuming protean proportions. It is becoming increasingly common to hear women complain of the sexual coldness, distance, and indifference of their dates, lovers, and mates. In a typical survey of college-educated young wives, 69 percent were satisfied with the frequency of their sexual relations, 6 percent found them 'too frequent,' while 25 percent complained of the infrequency of their marital relations. The fact that one in four women, at least in this study, found their mates relatively disinterested in sex is no small complaint, and echoes what most psychiatrists are hearing in their consultation rooms. Penile performance is apparently becoming perfunctory."

If surveys and polls can be relied upon, then they are telling us that Harry L. is part of a very rapidly increasing minority. In the 1940s, Kinsey reported that fewer than two percent of males under age thirty-five suffered impotence. By comparison, a 1970 survey by *Psychology Today* showed that more than one in every three men who responded was having erectile problems. Probably both surveys were inaccurate to a degree—in Kinsey's day only the rare man would have the courage to admit that he was impotent. And today we are too busy to fill out questionnaires unless the problems pertain to us personally. Even so, the variation in the two surveys is too radical to be that easily explained.

Says Kaye, "While statistics are readily available, quantifying the prevalence of influenza, divorce, heart disease, and unemployment in men, there is no agency that collects data on the incidence of impotency. Yet it is probably the case that impotency has become the least publicized epidemic of the past decade. This impression is gleaned from my patients, both male and female, from articles appearing in medical journals, and from conversations with my colleagues."

Erectile impotence is simply the inability to have an erection when it is wanted. Obviously, virtually every man has experienced impotence. The most robust twenty-year-olds, sexually aroused even after two or three orgasms, will find themselves incapable of attaining another erection immediately, however much they may theoretically desire one. That is certainly temporary "impotence."

Yet the word is a very poor one in the sexual context. Dictionaries tell us that "potent" means (1) powerful, mighty; (2) cogent, as reasons, etc.; (3) producing powerful physical or chemical effects, as a drug; (4) exercising great moral influence. Only the fifth and final definition makes reference to a lack of sexual power.

The point is that the word "impotent" cannot be used apart from the context of its major meanings. When we speak of impotence, we think of feebleness, scrawniness, canes, and wheelchairs, hopeless, helpless, deteriorated wrecks. Far preferable is a term such as sex dysfunction, preferred by William Masters and Virginia Johnson, authors of the landmark *Human Sexual Response.*

Sex dysfunctions develop for many reasons. Some few are physical. The twenty-year-old who has had a wild weekend of joyous debauchery and wants to make it just one more time to establish a new world record, and simply cannot, is probably experiencing either muscle fatigue or energy depletion. The diabetic who suffers circulatory complications may have erectile problems because the blood is not where it is needed when it is needed. Certain drugs can cause dysfunction. So can poor health. In some cases—not all, by any means—the body's efficiency decreases as it ages, and that can induce varying sexual incapacity. (We will discuss that fully in Chapter 9.)

Most dysfunction is psychogenic, however. That means it starts in the man's conscious mind. Perhaps he travels on business to a distant city, picks up a girl, takes her to his motel room. There, rather than relaxing into the sex situation, he thinks of his wife and children and starts feeling guilty. Suddenly he realizes he is not responding to the woman's caresses and her naked body. He panics at the awareness of his sudden incapacity to have sex. And that fear itself clinches his sexual dysfunction.

Another young man has always prided himself on being a sexual stud. One evening he dates a new girl. While petting her, he notes a particularly strong body odor. It offends him and suggests she is not particularly careful about cleanliness. Perhaps she even has venereal disease. The thought utterly destroys his sexual capacity.

A middle-aged man has been married twenty-five years and has always enjoyed sex with his wife. He has never had an extramarital relationship and never desired one. Now he is finding it more and more difficult to be "turned on" by his wife. His libido simply fails to be aroused by her, and she has mentioned the same lack of response. There is nothing new or refreshing in their sex lives. As a result, his erectile capacity has begun to flag.

In the sixteenth century the Arabian, Shaykh Nefzawi, referred to the "impossibility of coitus, owing to absence of stiffness in the member." He said,

> It will happen, for instance, that a man with his verge (penis) in erection will find it getting flaccid just when he is on the point of introducing it. He thinks this is impotence, while it is simply the result, maybe, of an exaggerated respect for the woman, maybe of a misplaced bashfulness, maybe because one has observed something disagreeable, or on account of the unpleasant odor; finally, owing to a feeling of jealousy, inspired by the reflection that the woman is no longer a virgin, and has served the pleasures of other men.

Nefzawi's certain cure: "They should eat stimulant pastry containing honey, ginger, pyrether, syrup of vinegar, hellebore, garlic, cinnamon, nutmeg, cardamoms, sparrows' tongues, Chinese cinnamon, long pepper, and other spices. They will be cured by using them."

Such problems as these—psychogenic ones—explain 95 to 98 percent of all erectile dysfunction, and although a greater percentage of men are suffering such problems today than in the past, the problem is as old as recorded history. So are the solutions. For example, in the ancient Hindu *Kama Sutra*, Vatsyayana writes,

> If a man desires to increase his sexual capacity both for his own pleasure and to ensure his success among women, there are herbs and medicines which make this possible.
>
> For instance, a man can greatly increase his sexual prowess by drinking milk mixed with sugar, the root of the plant uchchata, pepper, and licorice. Also, milk in which the testicles of a ram or a he-goat have been boiled produces the same effect. The juice of hedysrum gangeticum, kuili, kshirika, sansifiria, and roxburhiana mixed with milk are also effective.
>
> The ancient writers affirm that if a man grinds the grain and root of the trapa beipinosa, kasurika, jasmin and licorice, and an onion; mixes the composition with milk, sugar, and ghee; then, after boiling the mixture, drinks it, he will be able to enjoy innumerable women without fatigue or a diminution of his powers.
>
> Rice, sparrows' eggs boiled in milk with ghee and sugar produces the same result as does sesame seeds dipped in sparrows' eggs mixed with the fruit of the trapa bispinosa, kaskurika and when boiled with milk mixed with ghee, sugar, whole wheat flour and beans.

After proposing several such lists, Vatsyayana adds a word of advice: "But above all, one should be very careful not to try any dubious experiments that could bring about the deterioration of the body."

In some cultures, even today, the preferred treatment is calf's brain. Elsewhere, the impotent eat octopus, mice, eels, and ants. The Chinese depend on bird's nest soup. The ancient Romans ate the penises and testicles of horses and goats. In the civilized West, uninformed interest seems to have settled upon so-called Spanish fly (cantharides). Used in animals as a sexual stimulant for breeding, cantharides works not by increasing libido but by irritating the genitourinary tract. Sometimes the irritation can be severe enough to cause damage to the tissues. And in humans, according to Dr. Edward C. Muecke of the Departments of Surgery and Urology of the New York Hospital, "In both sexes, it [cantharides] can bring on breathing difficulty, coma, and ultimately death."

Muecke tells of a young man who took Spanish fly and came to the hospital two hours later, doubled over with abdominal cramps and nausea. Soon he broke out in blisters, suffered severe diarrhea, and vomited blood. He was compelled to urinate, but could do so only with great pain. Only emergency treatment saved his life.

Today many tabloids and girlie magazines carry ads for Spanish fly. The ads guarantee the products to be genuine. Perhaps they are—the household variety, captured, killed, and imported from Spain. They are not cantharides, which is a beetle, not a fly, under strict government control. It cannot be purchased even by prescription.

Right now aphrodisiacs, like the fountain of youth and Santa Claus, are pleasant pipe dreams. There is only one exception. In women it is always effective; in men only sometimes so. Says psychiatrist and sex therapist Helen Singer Kaplan, MD, PhD, "Testosterone is a highly effective aphrodisiac for women, probably especially when the androgen-estrogen ratio has been on the low side." In men testosterone's effectiveness depends on the cause of dysfunction.

Harry L., the twenty-four-year-old "boy" who wrote the letter to an endocrinologist in the hospital where he worked, had a stroke of good fortune. Virginia Huffer, the physician to whom he wrote, understood and was concerned. First she saw to it that he received psychotherapy. Then she began him on a testosterone replacement program.

Two years later Harry L. had left boyhood behind forever. He had taken on all the physical characteristics of adulthood—a deeper voice, muscularity, body hair, and an enlarged phallus. For the first time in his life he began to seek dates, have sex fantasies about girls, and experience erections. He began masturbating.

At the time Dr. Huffer made her report, Harry L., although much more aggressive and self-confident, still felt inadequate in his relationship to women. He had not gone beyond kissing on dates. Yet Dr. Huffer was confident that with time and continued therapy he would develop adequate sexual competence.

Another of Huffer's patients was a forty-six-year-old business executive. Although he had been married for twenty years, he had not once had sex with his wife. Before the marriage he had explained his lack of libido, and apparently she found the idea of marriage without sex perfectly satisfying.

He sought Dr. Huffer's help because of excessive fatigue. She did a hormone analysis, discovered a very low testosterone level, and prescribed testosterone replacement therapy.

Says Huffer, during the second month of therapy,

> He had marked increase in sexual drive directed toward women. His wife could not understand, let alone accept his sexual interests. He became aware of sexual impulses toward many women and even toyed with the idea of having an affair with one. Also, he seriously considered visiting a prostitute. However, because of his own standards, he renounced these ideas. During this period he became markedly irritable, which was most unlike him. However, his general strength had increased and also he experienced a sense of well-being that he had not had for many years.

The man was dangling from the horns of a dilemma. He found himself literally lusting after women, prepared for the first time in his life to enjoy sex. Yet neither his conscience nor his wife would permit him the release he sought. Rather than continue being unfulfilled and irritable, he discontinued testosterone therapy and drifted contentedly back to his sexless existence.

Joseph J. Sobotka of Phoenix, Arizona, is another physician who treats men with erectile dysfunction. Among the many successes he has reported is that of a twenty-six-year-old who came to his office complaining that for more than six months he had been unable to achieve an erection and orgasm more than once every two weeks. As with all of his patients, Sobotka's first step was to check for the uncommon but serious ailments of which impotence might be a symptom—cancer, kidney disease, diabetes, and such. The man was given a complete physical examination and his medical history was taken.

Satisfied that the partial impotence was not resulting from any overt disease, Dr. Sobotka prescribed testosterone tablets, one a day for four weeks. During that time the man's six-month pattern was dramatically shattered. He recorded seven erections and seven orgasms during each of the four weeks.

Many authorities with excellent credentials challenge testosterone's effectiveness in curing erectile difficulties. They point out the awesome power of suggestion and claim it is this effect, rather than the hormone, which stimulates the return of sexual capacity. They say that testosterone works as a placebo—a pill or capsule with no medicinal effect but which sometimes renders a cure through the power of suggestion. (It has been said the placebo is the most effective drug in the physician's pharmacopoeia.)

Dr. Sobotka anticipated the placebo argument, and so he took careful steps to answer it. After four weeks on testosterone therapy, he took the young man off all medication. Predictably, he promptly returned to an average of one erection and orgasm every two weeks. Then Dr. Sobotka prescribed the placebo. In every respect it appeared the same as the testosterone pill. Only a pharmacist could have known that the new batch of pills contained nothing more than sugar and chalk. Throughout the month the young man experienced the expected placebo effect—he had two erections and orgasms a week, far fewer than on testosterone.

In all, Sobotka treated fifty men with testosterone. They ranged in age from twenty-six to seventy-three and all had suffered erectile dysfunction for at least six months. He excluded all patients who had received any other form of treatment during the month before his study began in order to still the claim that credit for effectiveness might not belong to testosterone. Then he divided the fifty men into two groups—one containing twenty-eight patients, the other twenty-two. Although the men in the first group did not know it, they received testosterone for the first four weeks; then, after a month without therapy, they received the placebo for the second four. The second group received the placebo first. That answered any arguments that the order in which the drug is given has a suggestive effect on the outcome.

In his first group Sobotka had a thirty-four-year-old man who had suffered psychogenic impotence for two years. During that time he had averaged less than one orgasm a week. On testosterone he averaged three; on the placebo, one. Another man, thirty-six, complaining of extreme fatigue, had known no erections for half a year but had four a week, accompanied by two orgasms, on testosterone. He did not respond to the placebo. Two more men, forty-six and thirty-five, both suffering from psychogenic impotence for at least six months, had averaged only one orgasm every two weeks. On testosterone therapy the older man had three orgasms a week; the younger had four. Under the placebo they experienced one and two orgasms respectively each week.

The study of the second group may have been prejudiced against testosterone because of negative suggestion. Men who have experienced neither erections nor orgasms for periods ranging from six months to three years, then continue to have no response to placebos, and then endure another month without response, are rather thoroughly conditioned against responding to testosterone. Yet the hormone continued to prove effective in the second group.

A forty-eight-year-old man who had not had an erection or an orgasm within a year, and who had not responded to the placebo, developed three erections and one orgasm a week on testosterone. Another man, a year older and with precisely the same problem, found himself producing five erections and two orgasms a week.

The testosterone was effective. About that there can hardly be a doubt. In the first group the entire twenty-eight men produced only six erections and four orgasms a week prior to treatment. Under testosterone they developed 67.5 erections, an improvement of 1,025 percent. They had 39.25 orgasms, an increase of 823 percent. During the four-week rest period the effects of testosterone decreased, but enough of the hormone apparently still saturated the men's bodies so that the erection/orgasm level was higher than before the study began.

When the placebo was given first, the number of erections increased from 3.25 to 11.25, or 246 percent. Orgasms increased 169 percent, form 3.25 to 8.75. As with the first group, sex activity plunged during the four-week rest period. When testosterone therapy began, the men were experiencing 4.25 erections a week. That improved to 49.5, a change of 1,065 percent. Orgasms increased from 3.75 to 23, an improvement of 513 percent.

Regardless of honest skepticism, findings such as these cannot be ignored. Further, Brooklyn, New York, physician Robert Margolis and colleagues reported in the April, 1967, issue of *Current Therapeutic Research* a survey involving 500 physicians who prescribed testosterone for impotence. Among them they treated 2,000 patients ranging in age from 20 to 86. Of those, 1,499 reported for treatment regularly for three weeks, and by the end of that period 17 percent reported excellent results, 35 percent good, and 32.4 percent fair. Only 15 percent felt there was no response.

Testosterone can justifiably be called an aphrodisiac. But in another sense testosterone is not an aphrodisiac at all, for sometimes it produces no effect (as in Margolis' 15 percent), not even the placebo effect. A 36-year-old man who had suffered psychic impotence for a year and a half showed no improvement on testosterone in Dr. Sobotka's study. Neither did the 28-year-old with the same problem, or the 71-year-old, or the 66-year-old, both victims of physical degeneration.

To state what should be obvious: Apart from its placebo effect, testosterone can cure impotence only in very specific circumstances. The most obvious, of course, is a frank testosterone deficiency. Harry L. illustrates that condition. So does Dick M. He is a good-looking, friendly, fun-loving twenty-three-year-old who looked like he was fourteen and did not mind in the least, until his draft board rejected him. He told physicians, "I was shook. I never thought anything was wrong with me!" He had never dated, but that did not seem to matter. "It just never occurred to me to ask a girl for a date." He was interested in cars and sports, held a good job, and was given regular promotions, and would probably have gone through life perfectly content had the draft board's examining physician not rejected him on grounds of physical immaturity.

Six months after he began testosterone therapy, he learned what a sex life was. He started to ask girls out on dates and petted because it was fun, although not necessarily stimulating at first. At home he had frequent erections, he began masturbating, and later ejaculating. Months later, while kissing a girl, he had a spontaneous erection and a "special" feeling. Thereafter, kissing alone produced orgasm. Today, because of testosterone, the man is married and living a fully satisfying sex life.

Although the rule stands that the hormone can help only when a natural deficiency exists, testosterone *has* cured erectile problems when there were no *obvious* signs of deficiency. There are at least two possible explanations. As nutritionists have long known, minor deficiencies often exist on what is called the subclinical level. That means that the deficiency is not sufficiently serious to cause recognizable problems. Yet, if continued year after year, the shortage can cause subtle adverse effects on the body's health.

Precisely the same subclinical deficiencies can occur with hormones. As endocrinologist C. Alvin Paulson explains, "It takes ten to twenty years after the onset of testicular androgen failure before the deficiency is obvious to clinical examination." Recognizable deficiency usually occurs in the fifties so that subclinical shortages could begin in the thirties. If, during all those years, a man suffered subclinical deficiency, although there would be no overt, recognizable signs, he may well experience some difficulty in maintaining erection, diminution in the amount of fluid ejaculated, difficulty in achieving orgasm, and such. These symptoms may occur long before the more obvious signs of testosterone deficiency would develop—loss of libido, body hair loss, chronic weakness and fatigue. During the subclinical phase, even a blood and urine testosterone test might indicate low normal, thus failing to confirm the deficiency.

In a case of this sort, where the deficiency is so small as to be unrecognizable by laboratory tests, yet the tissues of the essential sex organs suffer chronic slight understimulation, testosterone supplementation can be very effective in restoring full potency.

Secondly, although a man may have an adequate saturation of testosterone in his body, raising testosterone levels higher than normal may produce additional effects. Dr. J. H. Vogelman of the Orentreich Foundation for the Advancement of Science calls it the principle of maximum genetic expression. We will discuss it in detail later, but basically it is the theory that virtually none of us fulfills the maximum potential we inherit in our genes. With the proper stimulation at the proper time in our development we could grow taller, more muscular, more obese, perhaps even more intelligent. It may be that above-normal testosterone stimulation can raise the libido higher—to the maximum capacity to which the man is genetically programmed.

That is hypothetical. So is the possible link between subclinical deficiency and sexual dysfunction. But whether for either of these reasons or for others not yet suspected, there is no question that some cases—though not all, by any means—of both physical and psychic erectile problems can be cured by testosterone.

8

Cycles and Variations

The daily routine of our lives is so thoroughly dominated by machines and computers that, for those of us who prefer laughter to tears, it seems grimly humorous. Filling out a credit application is a lengthy exercise in numerical recall: 249-70-2888 (Social Security number); 215-821-1960 (telephone number); 18102 (zip code); 5267-6312-060355 (credit card number); Q63AW (automobile registration); driver's license number; voter's registration number; draft board number and so forth, and so on and on and on.

Machines, not people, record the fact that we have or have not reported to work. Machines print our paychecks, send us overdue bills, argue with us when we have paid them, tell us when to drive and when not to, when to cross streets, and whether or not we should be permitted to die.

Man himself is rapidly being absorbed into this computer-mechanical universe, becoming another highly complex computer with an amazing knack for servicing, repairing, and maintaining itself, and whose primary function is to keep other computers and machines functioning and producing efficiently.

But, the fact is, man resembles a computer far less than he does the vast, rolling oceans, the clouds and wind, and the forests and wild animals. The skyscrapers and highways and the rockets and ocean liners are not his offspring but his creation. Unlike his hardware, man does not function in a steady state. He is a part of nature and, like all nature, the activities of his body ebb and flow rhythmically.

His hair growth is not a continuing process but occurs in spurts. He sleeps and awakens in cycles. His blood pressure, heart rate, respiration, urination, and defecation all follow cycles of their own. Our moods and behavior change. Some mornings we awaken optimistic; others we greet with gloom. We have good days and bad days, energetic ones and fatiguing ones. We will go for days being the most clear-minded, most quick thinking, and most decisive members of the species. A day or a week later we will curse ourselves for our thick-headed muddle-mindedness.

We do not function as machines but as entities of nature, in rhythms and cycles. And that is as true of our sex lives as of any other aspects of our existence. The first evidence of that resulted from animal studies some years ago. Researchers learned that male rabbits, cattle, mice, rats, and sheep produce varying volumes of ejaculate, have fluctuating levels of fertility, and produce more or fewer sperm, according to definite cycles. Even the sex drive in animals is cyclic.

The fact that the human female follows a distinct sex cycle is not a particularly original observation. But findings of a study at Cornell College in Mount Vernon, Iowa, extend the implications of the menstrual cycle to suggest that even sexual desire may be rhythmic, perhaps a remnant of the primitive "heat" phase of other species. The Cornell College study involved forty-eight women—dormitory residents eighteen to twenty-two years old. Each viewed photographs of handsome young men in suits, coats, and swimming trunks. The photos they found of no interest they rated number one. Those very stimulating they rated five. They rated the others between the two extremes. The test was administered twice, first on the fifteenth day of each girl's menstrual cycle, presumably when most of them were ovulating. At that point women are most susceptible to impregnation. The test was given a second time two weeks later.

The researchers concluded: "The ovulating woman is more

likely than the premenstrual woman to describe herself as responsive to sexually-arousing stimuli." In practical terms: Most women reach a peak of sexual desire about two weeks after they begin menstruation. If a woman is usually reticent regarding sexual activity, she will be more positively inclined to sex advances at that time. If she is naturally sexually permissive, she may very well become the aggressor during ovulation. According to another study, published in *Nature* (November 9, 1968), "The rates of intercourse and orgasm at one point in the cycle (during ovulation) are from two to six times the rate at other points in the cycle." Thus a woman is likely to desire sex at least twice as frequently, and perhaps six times so, during ovulation, as compared to her normal levels of desire.

Sex interest cycles also seem to relate to pregnancy in women. Findings by Masters and Johnson indicate that women become increasingly interested in sexual activity during the second three months of pregnancy. During the last three months, obviously, because of the added weight burden and discomfort, sex interest wanes.

Far more time and money have been invested in understanding female sexual cycles than male, but recent research shows that men, too, have sexual cycles similar to those found in animals. Investigators at the Kobe University School of Medicine in Kobe, Japan, took blood samples from twenty healthy young men every second day for two months and found that blood testosterone levels fluctuated widely during that time (from 14 to 42 percent, obviously an enormous variation). More than half the men followed clearly discernible testosterone-producing cycles. Some were as short as eight days, but most fell within the twenty- to thirty-day range, which led the researchers to conclude that, "the average cycle length may approximate that of the female menstrual cycle."

The effect these cycles produce in men is still undetermined. In only one case was a definite link found between peak testosterone levels and maximum sex drive and activity. One possible reason, according to researcher Charles H. Doering, of the department of psychiatry at Stanford University School of Medicine, is that testosterone in the *blood* is not necessarily testosterone available to the *body*.

That is an important point. Most testosterone does *not* flow freely in the blood of either men or women, but binds with a protein called sex hormone binding globulin (SBG). Until it is released from the SBG, the hormone cannot be utilized; only the one to three percent that is "free" can produce any psychophysiological effects. Perhaps *free* testosterone levels are completely unrelated to *total* hormone levels. The sex hormone binding globulin (SBG) itself may well have a cycle of its own, and until that can be measured, the male "monthly" sex cycle will remain theoretical.

Another possibility Doering suggests is that "additional behavioral measures would reveal a closer relationship between the fluctuation of circulating hormones and mood and behavior than we have been able to demonstrate." Perhaps there *are* changes in mood and sex interest during the testosterone production cycle, but the myriad distractions of our typical everyday life-style suffocate spontaneous response. Only through much more sophisticated tests than are now available will subtle variations in sex interest from day to day be identified.

Men also apparently have an *annual* sex cycle, which may explain the fact that there is a consistent rise in conceptions in September and October each year and a low point in the spring. Presumably people enjoy sex year-round. Yet as spring approaches each year, fertility declines.

An explanation based on studies with Japanese quail is suggested by Wilbur O. Wilson, PhD, of the department of avian sciences, University of California at Davis. Wilson divided the birds into two groups. One was kept at a constant 50° F temperature; the other at 90°. After four weeks all the quail were killed. The testes, or ovaries and oviducts, were weighed. Said Wilson, "Autopsies revealed that the weights of the gonads from these trials were significantly larger in the hot than in the cold environment."

If that research can be adapted to humans, it implies that sperm and testosterone production during the winter months decrease along with the size of the testes, and that might have a libido-reducing effect. Perhaps that is the reason we tend to associate the tropics and warmer climates with sensuality and eroticism.

Two additional testosterone production cycles have been identified in man; one is daily and the other is in minutes. The daily cycle has been proven many times, most recently by Robert Rubin of the Max Planck Institute for Psychiatry in Munich. In careful studies he showed that the testosterone levels were highest between two and four A.M. At their peak, levels may be two or three times that of their lowest point, apparently around eleven P.M. or midnight.

Another study, at Montefiore Hospital in New York City, suggests that high testosterone levels continue through the after-breakfast hours of the morning. But by eleven A.M. a significant decrease develops and continues through midafternoon. The drop from eight thirty A.M. to three P.M. is more than forty percent.

Nearly all birds and most animals mate during the daylight hours, and it may be that man, too, is predisposed to daytime sex. Commonly, young men awaken with erections, often not caused by the pressure of a full bladder. Future research may reveal that it is nature's way of telling us that morning sex is physiologically more desirable. Traditionally our sex lives have been crushed into the organized machinery of our life-styles. Rather than taking the time and trouble to undress and go to bed twice a day, we simply set sex aside until the late evening hours, finally coming to it with bodies and minds exhausted beyond passion, devoid of the energy to experience the delights of pure, wholesome lust, satisfied to score for scoring's sake—if we can manage even that.

The recent discovery of a very short-term testosterone cycle came about through painstaking research at the University of Texas. Keith D. Smith, MD, with the medical school's Program in Reproductive Biology and Endocrinology, hired four men to do nothing but relax on couches for eight hours while, every two minutes, he withdrew a small amount of blood through a hollow needle in their arms. The result: dramatic fluctuation of testosterone levels for each of the men. But the durations of cycles varied greatly. For some they were only four minutes; for others an hour.

That finding is more than a curiosity. It illustrates how little we know and how much there is yet to know in the young science of endocrinology in general, and about the male hormone in particular. We do not know whether those fluctuations have any importance physiologically or psychologically. But we *do* know that we cannot depend on a once-and-done test to determine a man's testosterone level. Depending on when, in the minute-to-minute cycle, the blood sample is taken, it may show very low production levels or very high, although over a twenty-four-hour period the man may produce a perfectly normal amount of hormone. Yet, virtually all physicians testing testosterone levels will take one and only one blood sample. Except in extreme deficiency or excess, such tests reveal little.

But let us presume two men are subjected to the same detailed tests. Barry is well-built and has heavy hair growth on his chest and legs. His voice is deep, his manner masculine. Paul is taller than Barry, but lean and scrawny. Except for the pubic area and underarms, his body is hairless. Yet several tests show that Paul has a higher testosterone production rate than Barry!

The reason is, in Roger Williams' words, "biomedical individuality." In his book by that name, Williams explains that normal testes have been found to vary in weight from 10 to 45 gms. (In fact, atrophied testes may weigh as little as a half gm.) A logical assumption is that larger testes will contain more interstitial cells and thus produce more testosterone. And that seems to be the case. In fact, Williams suggests that there is an eleven-fold range in daily testosterone production in normal men—some men producing 20 IU and some as much as 225 IU daily.

Because of his biochemical individuality, Barry's body may function with great efficiency on perhaps 100 IU of testosterone. Paul's body, however, is not an efficient testosterone user. Perhaps it lacks what is called end-organ responsiveness—the tissues needing the hormone respond to it more sluggishly than they should. Although he may produce 175 IU or more daily, much of it is wasted. Another possibility: His system may produce excess sex hormone binding globulin (SBG), which we mentioned earlier. No matter how much testosterone he produces, it is held captive by SBG and cannot meet the body's needs.

Still another possibility: Paul's testes secrete more estrogen than Barry's do. Normal males vary widely not only in their testosterone production, but also in the production of estrogen. Thus Williams suggests classifying men sex-hormonally according to nine groupings. "Placing the androgen (all male sex hormones, including testosterone) production first and the estrogen production second, these groups are: (1) low-low, (2) low-intermediate, (3) low-high, (4) intermediate-low, (5) intermediate-intermediate, (6) intermediate-high, (7) high-low, (8) high-intermediate, and (9) high-high."

According to that classification, Barry may have been an intermediate-low and Paul a high-high. Estrogen, remember, is in a sense the enemy of testosterone in the system, competing with it for carrier proteins and enzymes needed for conversion to active forms, and apparently even going so far as to tell the hypothalamus to stop ordering testosterone production.

Where do *you* fit in the nine groups? Unless you have seriously hyperactive or inactive testes, no simple blood or urine testosterone level test can answer that question. Yet few doctors go beyond those simple tests. Thus when they assure their patients that their testosterone levels are perfectly adequate, the physicians may be unintentionally misinforming them.

Before that assurance can be justifiably made, at least one more test is required. We have mentioned repeatedly that the testes must be stimulated by two hormones from the pituitary gland before they will do their work of producing sperm and testosterone. Testing for these two pituitary hormones (interstitial cell-stimulating hormone and follicle-stimulating hormone) can tell a knowledgeable physician a great deal. If they are present in large quantities, the physician knows there is not enough testosterone in the blood to reach the pituitary and curtail its hormone secretion. On the other hand, if there is no pituitary gonadotrophic hormone in the blood, chances are good that there is sufficient testosterone present to meet the body's needs and turn off pituitary gonadotrophin secretions.

Even that test is not infallible. A diseased pituitary could become either hyperactive or inactive. Except for that rare possibility, however, the test can be relied on, for pituitary gonadotrophin secretions are dependent upon one's own individual testosterone needs, cycles, and variations. Like all testosterone tests, the pituitary gonadotrophin test should be given several times to account for cyclic differences. It is the only way to be certain whether or not you are suffering a testosterone deficiency.

9

Aging—Why Bother?

Every day five thousand Americans reach their sixtieth birthdays. Often it is a time of less than heartfelt celebration. Birthdays highlight what Nathan W. Shock terms the physiology of aging, the step-by-step deterioration of the body over a course of years which, until recently, appeared to represent the irrevocable destiny of us all. Today gerontological researchers have begun to think of aging as a disease—perhaps several diseases—rather than a natural occurrence. They have made great strides in understanding its causes, both on the cellular level and that of the total body organism. Pioneer investigators around the world are treating elderly men and women in many ways undreamed of a decade ago, sometimes with extraordinary results. One of the gerontologist's most effective weapons in the campaign against aging in elderly men is testosterone.

Under ordinary circumstances, after the age of 26 the body literally and inexorably deteriorates:

—Between 35 and 80, the capacity to do physical work falls almost 60 percent.

—By 75 years of age the brain weight has decreased by 44 percent, and that organ receives 20 percent less blood than it did in young adulthood.

—Cardiac output is reduced by 30 percent.

—The number of nerve trunk fibers, which account for one's

capacity to respond to stimuli, is decreased by 35 to 40 percent.

—Taste buds die off, so that the elderly have only one third as many as a 30-year-old.

—There is only about half the capacity for oxygen utilization there once was.

—The heart works harder to pump more blood.

—Reflex responses and decision making require more time.

—Respiratory function, the amount of oxygen the lungs can process, declines by about 40 percent.

—Between the ages of 35 and 80 the flow of blood plasma through the kidney declines by 55 percent. As a result, the kidneys take a good deal longer to do their job.

—Hormonal output diminishes.

—In the words of Nathan Shock, "A key characteristic of aging is a reduction in the reserve capacities of the body—the capacities to return to normal quickly after disturbance in the equilibrium."

Additionally, there are the myriad aches and pains, and discomforts and inconveniences of aging—the decline in hearing capacity and eyesight, the reduced bladder control and capacity, the dry, wrinkled skin, the shrinking and weakening muscles, the stiff and swollen joints.

Sexual changes occur, too. Some individuals refer to them as evidence of a male menopause, a biologically absurd attempt at unisexual nonsense.

The changes that occur in *some* men with age, often called the climacteric, trouble a minority, variously estimated at 15 to 35 percent. It usually occurs in men between the ages of 48 and 60, slightly later than in the female. About 20 percent of men between 48 and 58 experience the climacteric, and about 30 to 35 percent between the ages of 58 and 68.

Changes in thinking and attitude are among the early indications of approaching climacteric. A man who may have been very decisive early in life may begin pondering the smallest problems, vacillating rather than committing himself to a position. He will lack self-assurance or flounder in situations where he would in earlier years have taken complete control. Even when he knows he has a good idea, he will lack forcefulness to push it through. But the good ideas will come far less frequently—he will be convinced that somehow his mental alertness is flagging.

So is his physical strength. Sometimes his heart beats irregularly, which frightens him. He has dizzy spells, heat flashes which at night sometimes keep him awake. No wonder he is irritable and difficult to live with. He knows it but he is helpless to change.

The most important differences in his life are sexual, and they may well account for some of the others. The typical man past fifty is not having as much sex as before. Whereas he may have had two orgasms a day in his twenties, he is satisfied with two a week now. Masters and Johnson, after interviewing 212 men more than fifty years old, report they "find that they cannot redevelop penile erections for a matter of twelve or twenty-four hours after ejaculation." Three decades earlier, these same men may have produced second erections within moments of ejaculation. Some young men, in fact, maintain an erection through two orgasms.

The older men also do not frequently experience rapid erection. It may take fifteen minutes or more of foreplay, sometimes involving rapid frictional stimulation of the genitals, before the penis is prepared for coitus. The orgasm itself may be of shorter duration—4 to 8 seconds in younger men and 2 to 4 seconds in men beyond 50. The quantity of ejaculate will be about 2 cc's, as compared to 5 cc's in men less than 40 years old.

One obvious explanation for some of these changes seems to have been given little if any attention: After thirty-five or forty years of orgasms, some men simply become a bit bored with sex. (Some women report such attitudes much earlier in life.) Unlike eating and sleeping, sex is not an *essential* biological drive. Even the most sexually active men will completely lose interest in sex if they are preoccupied with any number of other interests. Fear, hunger, depression, fatigue, intense concentration, or curiosity—these are but a few factors that can and do take precedence over the sex drive.

The mind of a man in his fifties is often cluttered with a great many pressing problems and questions, not the least of which is his own mortality. These are distractions against which the pleasant but utterly familiar sensations of a naked body against his own simply cannot compete.

Says Robert N. Butler, MD, psychiatrist and gerontologist, "The common causes of loss of sex drive are depression, anxiety, anger, performance anxiety, boredom, fear of a heart attack," all psychological distractions. To that list Butler adds only four physical causes of sex drive loss: drugs, poor physical fitness, obesity, and diabetes.

Apart from those physical factors, then, decreasing sexuality with age is, at least on the surface of it, a result of preoccupation with negative thinking. And that in itself is another symptom of aging.

For more than a quarter of a century now a handful of pioneering physicians have been treating their aging patients with testosterone. Originally the goal was primarily to restore sexual functioning. But adequate doses of the drug for prolonged periods have done much more, according to the practitioners, restoring many of the physical and psychological characteristics of young and middle-aged men.

One veteran testosterone therapist is Thomas Reiter, MD, of Berlin. Writing in the *Journal of the American Geriatrics Society*, Reiter told of some of his experiences with 240 elderly men he treated with testosterone implants. In one case a sixty-year-old man came to his office and reported total impotence for the previous two years. He suffered severe depression and was particularly troubled that he could not sleep throughout the night, but had need to rise frequently to urinate. Reiter prescribed testosterone. Within three months the man's sexual capacity returned to normal. According to Reiter, "Depression and lassitude changed to exuberance and a great deal of new activity."

Reiter described another case: "A.P., age sixty-nine, consulted me regarding impotence, depression, and inability to concentrate. Retirement from a heavy and responsible job seemed necessary, and depressed the patient greatly. Urinary symptoms were very marked."

The man was given regular and increasingly more potent doses of the hormone. Nine years after the therapy began, Reiter wrote, "His potency is still good. He personally conducts all business activities and assumes the heavy responsibilities of his firm. Now at the age of seventy-seven he is a happy, cheerful man who is willing to carry on."

Reiter's rating scale, by which he measures his patients' improvement, includes values for impotence, depression, and urinary disturbance. Regarding impotence, patients are classified from 12 to zero. Complete impotence of at least two years' duration scores 12. The man's presumed potency at age 25 rates zero. The depression is similarly rated—normal is zero and the severest neurotic disturbance is 8. The urinary disturbance scale rates severe frequency and urgency during the daytime and at least three nightly micturitions at six. Normality again is zero.

Reiter evaluated every one of his 240 patients before testosterone therapy, two months after treatment began, and four months after. In some cases the results were minimal or nonexistent. In others the improvement was dramatic, especially when higher doses were used. A 52-year-old whose rating was 12-8-5—total impotence, severe depression, and serious urinary difficulties—became a 5-3-2 within four months. He reestablished the sexual behavior of a man in his thirties, suffered no more depression than most of us do, and almost completely overcame urinary problems.

A 65-year-old dropped from a 12-7-5 to a 5-5-3. A young man aged 40, originally a 10-6-2, improved to a 4-3-1. An Army major aged 63 dropped from 12 to 7 on the potency scale.

In some cases the potency scale improved but the depression did not. In others the results were reversed. Reiter had no means of predicting who would be helped, how much, and in what way. But his lengthy tables and charts leave no doubt that androgen therapy arrests or reverses at least some symptoms of aging in a significant number of older men.

New York City endocrinologist Herbert Kupperman, MD, has been prescribing testosterone therapy for many years. He says:

> There's usually improvement within six weeks. We see the return of potentia (sexual capacity), a reduction in depression—in general, a reduction of all the symptoms associated with the climacteric.
>
> If a patient has a good response, I intermix placebo injections about two months into therapy and continue those injections for a couple of months. If he notes a change for the worse, I have another means of proving that what I was giving him was of some help and immediately start him back on the real drugs.

Another who uses the placebo test is the eminent obstetrician Dr. Robert Greenblatt. In case after case, within a few days or a week after receiving the placebo, his patients have returned to him to say, "Something is wrong, Doctor. The drug is no longer working."

Miley B. Wesson, MD, of San Francisco has been prescribing testosterone therapy since 1932. In his experience he has found that "testosterone used in adequate dosage over a long period of time can result in striking, even 'miraculous,' improvement in muscle tone and a general sense of well-being. It can act like a tonic, making old men 'young,' and young men more vigorous sexually." Among the case histories in his files is the following:

> Following World War II, a 61-year-old Vice-Admiral (retired because of age) was sent to me because he was very desirous of marrying a beautiful 28-year-old Navy nurse. For several years he had lived a continent life and was completely impotent. He had explained his condition to her, and she, being very much infatuated with the old gentleman, said she was willing to live an asexual life with him. He was referred to me by his lawyer, a woman superior court judge who, while in my office, overheard me talking to a patient. I advised 50 mg of testosterone intramuscularly twice a week. This schedule was continued for some time with testosterone that he obtained free from the Navy dispensary. Recently he brought his family to show me. There are now three children, ranging in age from six to ten years. (His wife told me that she never failed to use her diaphragm because her family is large enough.) Incidentally, he has not a wrinkle in his face and is active in business, having established a very lucrative insurance agency.

The male climacteric is not merely the series of symptoms we have been discussing. It is, in Dr. Kupperman's words, "that stage in a man's life when gonadal function diminishes, eventually resulting in complete cessation." Many of the physical, sexual and psychological symptoms of the climacteric may grow out of that one central fact—decreasing testicular function.

Men from 72 to 90 years old will produce only 42 percent of the testosterone they did between the ages of 23 and 39. And researchers are not sure that even that limited amount is entirely utilized. In recent years investigators have undertaken intensive research to explain precisely why testosterone levels decrease in aging men.

As we've found with the hypothalamic-pituitary-gonadal axis, the body's endocrine functions are circular—the level of one influencing the level of another, and then another, which finally controls secretion of the first hormone. Ultimately something in that circle changes, causing a subtle and prolonged decrease in testosterone production. Researchers are hungry to know where to break into the circle, what is the "first cause" of decreasing efficiency of the testicles. For now the starting point must be arbitrary, based more on hunches than on demonstrated fact.

One beginning might be with the blood supply to the testicles. Since the early nineteen sixties, statements attributing hundreds of thousands of deaths each year to arteriosclerosis and related diseases have created widespread awareness of this illness. In arteriosclerosis the blood vessels, ordinarily rubbery, grow brittle. The inside walls thicken, and in a particular type of arteriosclerosis—atherosclerosis—fatlike gobs accumulate along the vessel walls, partially blocking blood flow. Around these gobs, called plaques, blood sometimes pools and forms a plug that completely blocks the vessel. That is known as a thrombus or thromboembolism. If the thrombus develops in a vessel carrying blood to the heart for its nourishment, a coronary thrombosis, or a potentially fatal heart attack occurs. In the brain the blockage causes a stroke.

As long as these blockages are only partial, they cause no pain and often go undetected. Indeed, most of us undoubtedly have some degree of arteriosclerotic disease already. Two studies performed on young men killed in action during World War II revealed advanced arteriosclerosis in a significant number—this among men aged eighteen to twenty-two years old!

Arteriosclerosis may affect many or all of the body's blood vessels. That includes those nourishing the testicles. A decreasing blood supply means less oxygen and fewer nutrients available to the cells. Some cells die. Those that live are less healthy than normal. When the blood supply to a certain area of the heart is blocked, the muscle tissue thus starved dies, and the heart must either collapse or function with the impairment. When blood is blocked to the brain, cerebral cells quickly starve from oxygen lack, often causing irreparable or fatal damage. Logically, plaque blockage of the tiny blood vessels nourishing the testicles could in itself cause their malfunction in later years.

In fact, preliminary research supports that idea. The testes do become smaller in old age. Cells that compose them, including the interstitial cells, die. Only those in close proximity to the blood vessels and capillaries survive. The areas in the testes where the losses are greatest are those farthest removed from the blood supply. As the interstitial and seminiferous cells die, sperm and testosterone production decreases. The hypothalamus and pituitary, heavily supplied with large blood vessels, do not suffer this deterioration. The pituitary continues to send gonadotrophins, interstitial cell-stimulating hormone, and follicle-stimulating hormone to the testes. And the testicular cells that remain do their best to follow instructions. There are simply not enough left.

Drawing on some of the facts we have discussed in earlier chapters, we can almost predict the next step in the circle. While testosterone production decreases, that of the sex hormone binding globulin (SBG) does not. In fact, some researchers feel SBG production actually increases with age. Whether or not this is true, the results are still the same: Virtually all the meager testosterone produced in the aging man is bound with the globulin, leaving none free in the bloodstream to reach the cells of the sex organs and thus meet the body's needs. Estrogen, however, does not bind as well to SBG, so estrogen levels continue to rise in the blood. By impersonating testosterone, the female hormone gets absorbed in place of testosterone when the latter is not available, and this leads to feminization.

There is apparently no doubt among physicians that in men whose testes are not producing adequate levels of testosterone (called hypogonadal men), testosterone can prove extremely therapeutic. It does not matter if these patients are fifteen, fifty, or seventy years old. But frequently a man suffering symptoms of the climacteric does not show a clearcut deficiency of testosterone. As we have already explained, hormones are very potent substances with far-reaching effects throughout the body, and most physicians prefer not to prescribe replacement therapy for a hormone that does not need replacement.

As a rule involving drugs in general, that attitude is honorable. Far too many drugs are prescribed far too casually in this country. Regarding testosterone therapy, however, the following questions arise:

1. Has the patient been tested not only for blood and urine testosterone levels but also for pituitary gonadotrophin? Without the pituitary tests there is no assurance that testosterone levels are adequate, no matter what the blood and urine tests show.

2. Have the tests been repeated several times to offset cyclic variations?

3. Is there reason *not* to prescribe testosterone, i.e., is the patient suffering prostate cancer? With the possible exception of a capacity to exacerbate an already existing cancer of the prostate, testosterone is viewed by physicians as a relatively harmless substance which, in excess, is broken down and eliminated from the body in the urine. Unlike some other hormones (insulin, for example), testosterone is potent in doing its job of masculinizing the body, but is harmless in men in excess.

4. Sometimes the symptoms of aging can be alleviated by the male hormone even when tests fail to show a testosterone deficiency. One recent example of that comes from researchers at the Worcester, Massachusetts, State Hospital. Psychiatrists there cured eight elderly male patients of depression through high doses of testosterone, although they showed no frank testosterone deficiency.

The first step in treating sexual dysfunction and other symptoms of the climacteric in older men is the crucial matter of ruling out serious disease through a thorough physical examination for diabetes, heart disease, serious arteriosclerosis, and such. Early diagnosis and specific treatment of these maladies can save lives, and testosterone does not do the slightest good.

But where no specific illness exists, the advice of C. Alvin Paulson, MD, is as good as any. He recommends what he calls the "testosterone therapeutic test," a series of hormone injections administered daily for two weeks. Writing in Williams' *Textbook of Endocrinology*, he said, "One week after the cessation of therapy the patient is interviewed and the test is considered *positive* for Leydig (interstitial) cell failure if (1) amelioration of the 'climacteric' symptoms occurred slowly, i.e., near the end of the first week; and (2) the relapse was gradual after the injections were discontinued." Or, more simply, try it, and if it works, it proves a deficiency existed. Considering that testosterone is inexpensive, Paulson's "testosterone therapeutic test" appears to be the epitome of common sense once prostate cancer has been ruled out. The medical literature confirms extensively that hypogonadal men given testosterone experience clear-cut dramatic improvement and *know* a change has taken place.

Thus the circle that produces the climacteric can be broken through testosterone replacement. But recent research has uncovered another way the circle can be broken.

Some years ago it was discovered that the placenta surrounding the fetus in the mother's womb produced a particular hormone, human chorionic gonadotrophin (HCG). Since then, researchers have learned to synthesize HCG inexpensively in a laboratory from the urine of pregnant women, and investigators have conducted many experiments with it.

One thing they have learned is that HCG can function similarly to those pituitary hormones which stimulate the testes to produce testosterone—interstitial cell-stimulating hormone and follicle-stimulating hormone. Yet there is a difference. Human chorionic gonadotrophin (HCG) stimulates the interstitial cells to function *even in the aged*, which the pituitary hormones cannot do. In 1974, R. Rubens, a Belgian endocrinologist, and his associates reported in the *Journal of Clinical Endocrinology and Metabolism* that human chorionic gonadotrophin (HCG) stimulation caused an 85-percent increase in testosterone levels in men 65 and older. That same year Italian endocrinologist Dr. C. Mazzi reported even more significant results. He found that young men given massive doses of HCG had a 121-percent increase in testosterone production. And six elderly men, 72 to 90 years old, experienced a 110-percent increase. Under HCG they were producing testosterone at normal levels for men in their twenties.

A 72-year-old man increased testosterone production by 121 percent. An 81-year-old had a 157-percent increase. Another man, 82, improved 110 percent. And the 90-year-old increased testosterone levels by 69 percent.

No one is sure how human chorionic gonadotrophin (HCG) produces such results. Perhaps it stimulates the production of new interstitial cells. Or it may push the remaining old ones to greater production. Future endocrinologists may use HCG to enable aging men with testosterone deficiencies to regain their own testosterone-producing capacity, which would be less expensive and more convenient than chronic visits to the doctor for testosterone replacement therapy.

It is safe to say that not too long from now gerontologists, endocrinologists, psychologists and sexologists will emphatically agree that no healthy man, regardless of age, should be condemned to faltering testosterone levels. Testosterone as a drug is no less a miracle than is any other hormone—adrenalin, thyroxin, insulin. It is not a bit less magical than the vitamins and trace minerals. It is a substance normally found in the body, a chemical that belongs there. What is amazing is not the fact that, by replacing the hormone, vigor, sexual capacity, energy, and optimism can be restored. The puzzle is that relatively few aging men have been offered testosterone therapy.

There are several possible explanations for the hesitancy. For one thing, the old Brown-Séquard reaction still lingers. That is understandable for, along with cancer cures and vitamin supplements, the male sex hormone has been subjected to the claims and promotion of quacks. Whenever radical, unexpected, and unsubstantiated claims are made for a new drug or product, sincere medical practitioners almost inevitably are frightened away. Even a man of Charles Édouard Brown-Séquard's stature was scoffed and denounced when he spoke of sex gland therapy, and it is no wonder that patent medicine salesmen hawking sex hormone elixirs in the early decades of this century have succeeded in souring some physicians on testosterone's therapeutic value.

If some doctors considered testosterone little more than an ineffective patent medicine, others may be somewhat intimidated by a fear of side effects, particularly the idea held some years ago that testosterone may produce cancer of the prostate.

The matter cannot be dismissed by a cursory statement, and we have devoted an entire chapter to giving the full story. For now we will repeat what we have already said several times: Testosterone does not cause cancer. If cancer already exists, testosterone may enhance its growth, although some researchers doubt even that.

There may be another reason doctors do not more often prescribe testosterone, particularly for aging patients. It is a philosophical attitude rather than a medical one, the view that it is natural for all men to age, for their bodies to slow down, and their sex lives to wane. It is all part of life's inexorable deterioration. "Why fight nature?" is the pervasive philosophy. "Contentment for the aging man comes by facing the inevitable with sublime resignation, not by foolishly struggling to maintain youth."

Apart from the probable incapacity of the western mind to accept this nirvanalike psychic suicide, the attitude has a colossal weakness. Many aspects of the aging process *can* be slowed, and, as we have seen, may even be reversed with testosterone administration. We do not permit a man who has lived beyond fifty or sixty years of age to deteriorate with disease or with malnutrition if we can help it. It is time we began showing equal concern for the man deteriorating from hormonal insufficiency.

10

Making Muscle—and Keeping It

Even as a child Edward R. had been obese. For years he provided a favorite entertainment for other children in the neighborhood—teasing Eddie. Even adults chided him—his parents, the physical education teacher, the school nurse. A teacher once called him a pig.

Ed grew into his teenage years a master of the art of avoidance. He threatened to have himself expelled from school unless his parents persuaded the family physician to write a letter excusing him from gym. He joined no clubs and participated in no social activity. After school each day he promptly returned home, completed his homework, ate dinner, and watched television until bedtime. Ed never dated. He had considered it on occasion, and when he masturbated (once or twice a month), he fantasied being with a girl. But he refused to risk being rejected, so he simply avoided girls.

The most peculiar thing about Ed's obesity was his inability to explain it. For all the brutal remarks about his piggishness, he did *not* overeat. Once, in fact, he almost starved himself to death through a week-long crash diet. He did lose weight temporarily. Then he began eating again, a low calorie diet, and accompanied it with jogging and some push-ups. He could not exercise at any great length for he suffered excessive weakness, which the family physician shrugged off as a normal part of adolescence. Yet he pushed himself to the limits of his endurance. Still, for all his efforts, most of the weight returned as fat and not muscle.

Not until Edward R. was thirty-three years old did he finally discover the reason for his obesity.

Ken S. was exceedingly thin and equally weak, the original ninety-eight-pound weakling of those classic Charles Atlas ads. But no one kicked sand in his face at the beach for he was too ashamed of his emaciated appearance to expose himself to the world in a bathing suit. At age twenty-one he had already enrolled in a crash muscle-building program, had purchased a roomful of barbells and pressing equipment, and had swallowed gallons of every preparation on the market that promised to increase weight, muscle mass, or both.

None of it worked, not the protein-rich beverages, not the hour and a half daily training to exhaustion. Ken S. made one more investment. He visited an endocrinologist. Then he began building muscle.

George K., at the age of sixty-five, experienced a problem he had never faced in his life. He was growing weak. Even as a youngster he had been burly, tough. In high school he had been the county shot put champ and he had gone to college on a football scholarship.

Middle-age had not slowed him down. After work he visited the local YMCA every day, spent an hour jogging or swimming, and then walked home at a brisk pace. If his strength had been decreasing through the years, he had not noticed.

Then, during just the last few years, he suddenly recognized the change. His grip was not as strong. He could not run as long or as fast. He did not suffer rheumatism or any other common aches or pains of the aged. His muscles simply refused to perform. They grew fatigued more quickly than they did ever before.

He noticed another change, too. He awoke more frequently during the night with a compulsion to urinate. On two occasions he had not awakened soon enough. It left him feeling unspeakably disgusted with himself. Then George K. visited a gerontologist, and three weeks later he felt stronger—no

Superman, but obviously stronger. And the bladder problem had vanished.

Although each of these men had vastly differing symptoms, they suffered basically the same problem, insufficient testosterone to build and maintain muscle tissue.

Just as building contractors have their standard materials—steel, concrete, wood, glass, brick, and such—nature, too, has a standard set of building materials essential in constructing living bodies. They are called amino acids, and there are about twenty-one different kinds of them in nature.

Even plants are built from amino acids. They absorb nitrogen, carbon, hydrogen, and oxygen, and, by using the sun's rays for energy, convert them to amino acids. It is a neat trick. The plant literally builds its own body out of thin air. For its reward, the plant gets eaten.

It has to be that way, for most animals, including men, have not developed the knack for producing within themselves all the amino acids necessary for building their bodies. Instead, they acquire them by eating the plants that have produced them. A problem—no one plant produces *all* the essential amino acids ("essential" because man does not produce them in his body). Each plant specializes in a select few amino acids. Soybeans come closest to producing a full complement, but even they fall short.

There are two solutions. One could eat a wide assortment of fruits and vegetables, thus assuring himself of a fair sampling of amino acids. Alternatively, he may feed the plants to animals such as cattle. Fused in various combinations to build the plant's body tissues, the amino acids are called proteins. When the animal eats the plants, its digestive system breaks down the proteins into the basic amino acids once again. Carried through the blood to all the body's cells, these amino acids are once again assembled into the specific proteins needed by the cells. The protein becomes a part of the animal's muscle tissue, so that man can get his protein by eating meat. Meat has the major advantage of providing all eight essential amino acids. If a person had no other protein source but meat, he could continue to live and grow.

About 15 to 20 percent of our bodies is protein, about a third of which is in muscle and a fifth in bone cartilage. Protein exists in every cell. It is one of the components of enzymes, hormones, and body secretions. Hemoglobin, which in the bloodstream carries oxygen from the lungs throughout the body, is a protein. So are the antibodies which kill off invading bacteria. Skyscrapers are built of concrete, automobiles of steel, and people of protein.

A reasonable guess is that the man or woman who simply cannot build muscle must be suffering an amino acid deficiency. But that is not often true. Particularly in America authorities are more concerned that we are getting too much, rather than too little, protein. According to the Department of Agriculture, twice as much protein is available in our diets as is needed for adequate nutrition. In 1974, each American ate an average of 116 pounds of beef, an increase of 87 percent over the amount consumed 20 years ago. Each day many Americans eat three or four times the amount of protein their bodies can use.

Although most people do not realize it, protein, like carbohydrates and fats, is calorie-rich. In fact, both fats and protein contain four calories per gram. What's more, protein is a very adaptable nutrient. An excess of it can be used as an energy source. If it is not needed for that, it can also be stored as glycogen or adipose tissue, which means, of course, that too much protein can contribute to obesity. And today the typical American diet provides about 58 percent more protein than is needed for tissue building.

So it is not likely that men like Barry R., Ken S., or George K. are suffering amino acid deficiencies in their diets. But, just as a beach full of sand could not produce an ounce of concrete unless lime and cement were also present, so the amino acids are useless in muscle building unless additional substances are available.

Among these cofactors are hormones. Even an unborn baby's body is constructed largely from amino acids, and even then hormones are required. They are called *anabolic* hormones, those which permit living cells to convert the amino acids into human body tissue. (Incidentally, there are also *catabolic* hormones, which break down living tissues into their separate components.) In the fetus a hormone from the placenta, along with the testosterone in the male, stimulates protein-building growth. In the youth pituitary growth hormone (GH) is the major stimulus to muscle and bone building. But GH cannot work efficiently without the thyroid hormone, which is responsible for metabolizing GH and amino acids to cell tissue. People suffering thyroid problems frequently become obese, but not muscular.

As we said in Chapter 5, insulin, a powerful anabolic hormone supplied by the pancreas, is also an important contributor to childhood growth. Without it GH cannot function. But insulin is anabolic not only in terms of muscle, but also fat cells. That explains the fact that children usually have soft, undefined bodies, the muscle cells being generously interspersed with fat tissue.

Androgens, too, play a small part in childhood growth. Until puberty the adrenal glands of both girls and boys secrete the weak androgens known as 17-ketosteroid precursors. Throughout her life a woman depends upon the minute secretions of these substances and very minimal androgen secretions from her ovaries, along with the weak anabolic estrogen hormones, to build her body's musculature.

Incidentally, because the adrenals, the ovaries, or both are hyperactive androgen secretors in some women, or because they are actually pseudohermaphrodites with hidden testicles actively producing testosterone, those women are able to build much greater muscle mass than typical females. They easily excel in sports. Recently this has led to claims of unfair advantage by other competitors who insist that, beyond a point, the excess testosterone makes a female athlete no longer completely female and, in fact, perhaps more a man than a woman—in spite of external genitalia. The Olympic committee has heeded this complaint, and now requires female athletes to take a test to assure that they are genetic females.

The test, called a chromosome pattern analysis, was developed in the late nineteen fifties. Chromosomes are the substances in the genes which carry our hereditary information. As we have discussed earlier, normal females have two X sex chromosomes, while normal males have one X and one Y. If one of the sex chromosomes is either duplicated or deleted, the person does not follow a true male or female pattern.

The first woman to be banned from athletic competition on the basis of the chromosome test was a Polish sprinter twenty-one years old. In 1967 Ewa Klobukowska traveled to Russia to compete in track and field events but was disqualified following the test on grounds that genetic masculinity may indicate hidden testes or other sources of higher testosterone production than are found in normal women.

Although the woman relies primarily on the weak 17-ketosteroid precursors, the male at puberty begins producing testosterone. Most anabolic, or tissue-building, hormones work by increasing the number of cells, but testosterone is different. It enlarges the cells that already exist. And it does that with protein, converting it primarily to muscle and male sex organ tissue. When testosterone binds with amino acids, they are no longer available for energy, storage, and other uses. The body must then rely on carbohydrates and fats for those needs. That means that a normal teenage boy who does not overeat will tend to burn off his baby fat during his adolescent years and enter adulthood lean and muscular.

Unfortunately it does not always work out that way. Barry R. was as chubby an adult as he was a child. A very simple and inexpensive test helped to explain why.

About 16 percent of protein is nitrogen, so anyone with a chart giving the protein content of foods can easily calculate the amount of nitrogen in the food he eats. If the protein is absorbed into the body and used to build tissue, the amount of nitrogen secreted from the body in urine will, of course, be low. But if the body is not making use of the protein in the diet, the urine nitrogen content will be much higher. The nitrogen test today is dependable and its interpretation sophisticated. When a doctor speaks of positive nitrogen balance, he means that more nitrogen is being consumed in the diet than is being excreted—and that is good. The body is continuing to build tissue. If the intake/excretion levels are the same, that is not good. And if more nitrogen is being passed out of the body than is being taken in, muscle tissue is actually decomposing. That may occur when the body is calorie starved and is in urgent need of an energy source. It would prefer carbohydrates and fats, but if they are not available, the body will decompose healthy muscle tissue to convert protein to energy and excrete nitrogen as a waste product.

The breaking-down process—catabolsim—is, like anabolism, regulated by certain hormones. The most powerful catabolic hormone by far is cortisol from the adrenal gland. Excess thyroid hormone is also catabolic.

More detailed studies revealed relatively good news for Barry. Unlike some men with his symptoms, he did not have a hyperactive adrenal or thyroid gland. He suffered no serious disease. Only his testicles were malfunctioning—he produced insufficient testosterone. The doctor administered an injection of 250 mg of testosterone and told Barry to return in two weeks for another injection.

Imagine his elation—a man on the brink of middle age, scoffed and self-condemned all his life, shamed and guilt-ridden because of a grotesque body over which he had no control, rushing daily to the scales to prove the truth that his mirror told him. Within six weeks he lost twenty-three pounds according to the scale. But the *fat* loss was far more than that, for he had already begun adding muscle, which is three times as heavy as fat.

For the next six months Barry followed a special diet rich in sodium, chloride, potassium, phosphorus, and calcium, all minerals that combine with protein to form cell tissue. He also trained with weights three days a week to stimulate the buildup of additional muscle mass. In less than a year Barry, for the first time in his life, had a chiseled, rugged, athletic body.

Ken S. learned from his doctor what he had always suspected—that his testes were smaller than normal, softer, and almost nonfunctioning. The doctor's questioning reminded him that he had contracted mumps as a child and had suffered testicular pain for several days. The physician told him he had suffered mumps orchitis.

Barry and Ken suffered from basically the same problem—insufficient testosterone. Yet one was excessively obese, the other excessively thin. The explanation is as complex as the individual functions and myriad interactions of all the anabolic and catabolic hormones. To repeat the point: Each of us is unique. Some of us will react more radically to a testosterone deficiency than others will. A hyperactive thyroid or adrenal may burn fat from Ken, leaving only skin and bones, while sluggish endocrine glands in Barry may allow the adipose tissue to accumulate. Only elaborate tests can explain the great variation in response to testosterone deficiency.

Androgen replacement helped Ken gain weight almost immediately. Before treatment he excreted virtually all of the protein nitrogen he ate; afterward he retained virtually all of it.

To assure that the protein was used in building muscle rather than for energy or storage, Ken, like Barry, began to train with weights. He had another surprise. Prior to testosterone therapy, even exercise of short duration exhausted him. Now he found his endurance increasing significantly. He had greater energy output. The amount of weight he could lift improved weekly along with his muscle mass. Particularly the dimensions of his chest, biceps, and thighs increased.

Doctors would agree that Barry and Ken suffered from "official" physical ailments, but even in this day of medical advances some physicians would argue that the symptoms of a man George's age are the inescapable result of growing old. It is natural, they would say, for a man to grow weaker and less muscular with the overall deterioration we call aging.

In a sense they are correct. Writes the eminent gerontologist, Dr. Nathan Shock:

> Most of the debilities of age apparently result from a loss of tissue, particularly the death and disappearance of cells from the tissues. The wrinkled and flabby skin so apparent in elderly people offers mute testimony to this loss. Body weight declines, especially after middle age. In a large sample of male population in Canada average weight showed a decline from 167 pounds at 35 to 44 to an average of 155 pounds for men 65 and older. A sample of men in the United States, all of them 70 inches tall, averaged 168 pounds in weight at ages 65 to 69, and 148 pounds at ages 90 to 94. Women 65

> inches tall weighed, on the average, 148 pounds at ages 65 to 69, and 129 pounds at ages 90 to 94. . . .
>
> The microscope shows that in many tissues a decrease in the number of cells accompanies the weight loss. Connective tissue replaces the lost cells in some cases, so that the loss of cells is even greater than the reduction in weight would indicate. In the senile rat the muscle fibers showed degenerative changes with replacement by connective tissue and an increase in the spaces between fibers. Such loss of muscle fibers no doubt accounts in large measure for the lower muscular strength of elderly humans as well.

Ordinarily we are anabolic, or muscle-building, creatures in childhood, catabolic in old age. That fact alone explains many of aging's symptoms. A man who has lost muscle tissue cannot do as much work as before. He will utilize less oxygen to nourish fewer muscle cells. His heart—a muscle—will have a reduced work capacity; blood flow throughout the body diminishes, and that may have very far-reaching implications.

For example, reduced blood flow may be instrumental in the growing inefficiency of kidney function with age. Nerves, taste buds, brain cells, endocrine glands, and lung tissues all require rich oxygen supplies. Yet if the heart muscle weakens, it grows less and less capable of pumping oxygen-rich blood throughout the body. Theoretically, this chronic low-level oxygen starvation helps bring about the deterioration of essential body organs.

Perhaps a classic vicious circle develops. The blood supply to the testes decreases. That is known to reduce testosterone production. And that, in turn, permits further muscle, including cardiac, deterioration.

There is another way in which the normal decrease in testosterone production with age can lead to low-level oxygen starvation throughout the body. Testosterone is essential to the body's manufacture of red blood corpuscles, the cells that transport oxygen from the lungs to all parts of the body. If these cells are deficient, as they are when there is serious testosterone reduction, oxygen starvation is virtually inevitable. Even a quarter of a century ago many researchers recognized testosterone's value in treating angina pectoris, excruciating heart pain with feelings of suffocation and impending death, usually resulting from oxygen starvation of the heart muscle. In a great many cases testosterone relieved the symptoms and produced changes in the heart measurable on the electrocardiogram.

One consistent result of Dr. Reiter's work, discussed in the previous chapter, was improvement in bladder function and control. In case after case men who had poor urinary control improved, sometimes dramatically, after a few weeks on testosterone. Reiter himself suggested the increased bladder control may result from strengthened bladder muscles.

That same rationale may help to explain the improved sexual function in older men on testosterone therapy. Perineal muscles, located between the anus and the base of the penis, play a crucial role in the erectile mechanism. The weaker these muscles, the less turgid the erection. If the normal catabolic, or muscle-deteriorating, processes are reversed by testosterone, stronger erections could result.

Certainly testosterone therapy alone could never build or rebuild muscle. Certain enzymes must be present to decompose protein molecules. The protein itself must be available, along with the trace minerals we have mentioned. As we will see later, these substances may or may not be plentiful in an ordinary, well-balanced diet. Fish and chicken are preferable to beef and pork as protein sources since their fat content is much lower.

Muscle stress is another essential ingredient in serious muscle building, regardless of age. In effect, forcing muscle to its endurance limit notifies the body that more muscle mass is required. If there is no demand for increased muscle, the body will simply store or discard the excess protein.

So testosterone is not the whole answer to muscle building in the young, or combating the catabolism of aging. But it is an important aspect of the problem, and particularly in older men it holds great untapped promise. Says Dr. Reiter,

> We have reached a point where at last, by means of TI (testosterone implants, one of the methods of administering testosterone), we can take advantage of the full spectrum of

testosterone activity. This is of considerable practical importance, especially in the field of geriatrics. Nobody today considers the management of a diabetic problem without insulin. We may find in the future that nobody will consider the management of male geriatrics problems without testosterone implantation, unless some more effective method of clinical usage is developed.

11
Appearances

We recognize aging in ourselves and others not so much by what is happening internally as by the obvious external signs—the skin tells the story. When we say a man looks young for his age, we mean that his skin is tight and elastic, and when we say someone appears old beyond his years, we are usually referring to hanging and wrinkling skin. In desperation both men and women have sought to stop and even reverse the skin aging process, sometimes embracing bizarre, far-fetched, quackish, and expensive schemes. The "panaceas" have included mayonnaise, olive oil, tapioca, peaches and cream, the juice from melons, lemons, cucumbers, strawberries, and even green beans; eggs, honey, milk, cream, and buttermilk; oatmeal, almond meal, bran, and barley; coconut oil, castor oil, almond oil; animal fats, flour, and herbs.

Many older movie stars are said to have their favorites. Marlene Dietrich uses pure lanolin lotion on her face, neck, and hands. Joan Crawford applies wet tea bags to her eyes. The late Grace Moore, Metropolitan Opera star and actress, preferred castor oil. Gloria Swanson relies on raw fruit and vegetable for her face.

Unfortunately there is no reason to believe in the efficacy of any of these preparations, even among the great faces of yesteryear. Surgery—the face-lift—is, of course, a successful way of removing wrinkles, but it is not available to everyone because of the expense. And face-lifts are not permanent. If the skin continues to sag and age, additional operations are required to keep the skin tight. What's more, charlatans exist in the face-lift business just as they do in other fields. Many trusting people who have placed their faces in the hands of such incompetent practitioners still bear the scars to prove it.

Competent dermatologists have been searching for years for a way to control and perhaps reverse the skin's aging process. That was the reason why, more than a decade ago, Doctors Christopher Papa and Albert Kligman of the University of Pennsylvania School of Medicine in Philadelphia undertook some experiments with armpits! They sought to test their hypothesis that surface applications of the male hormone testosterone, if applied in large enough amounts and for a long enough period of time, could revitalize aging skin.

There was more to that study than appeared on the surface. No one would deny the psychological importance of a self-image. The man who finds a tired old face staring back from his mirror each morning may well feel defeated and without hope even before his day's work begins. Whether a man is seeking a promotion, a new position, or a new lover, or whether he just needs the assurance that he is simply in the ball park and playing the game, an aging face can be a serious handicap.

Even more significant: Old skin can have an adverse effect on the overall health of the body. Contrary to the general misconception, the skin is not simply a sack into which the body has been poured. It is an organ like the heart and lungs. In fact, it is the largest organ in the body, weighing about twice as much as the liver and totalling more than twenty-one square feet in most people. The skin is instrumental in keeping our inner temperature near 98.6°F, whether we are exposed to winter temperatures below zero or sauna heat above 200°F.

Antibodies and immune systems notwithstanding, the skin has the major responsibility for warding off infectious organisms. It removes wastes from our bodies, holds at bay environmental pollutants, sets up an impenetrable wall against the hundreds of chemicals we touch daily which, if absorbed into the blood, would certainly kill us. Bruised and scratched, burned and punctured, the skin is a tough, yet resilient, caressable fabric that might well leave the textile industry panting in envy.

Each square inch of that "sack" holding the body together contains:

78 nerves
650 sweat glands
19 or 20 blood vessels
78 sensory apparatuses for heat
13 sensory apparatuses for cold
1,300 nerve endings to record pain
19,500 sensory cells at the ends of nerve fibers
160 to 165 pressure apparatuses for the sense of touch
95 to 100 sebaceous glands
hairs and muscles
and 19,500,000,000 cells.

Actually there are two layers of skin. The surface layer, called the epidermis, is dead tissue, cells that have shriveled into tough flat plates somewhat resembling fish scales. The epidermis is the body's armor, and although it does not compete with the turtle's shell or a rhinoceros' hide, it still does a marvelous job. It keeps a bruise (bleeding beneath the skin) from developing into a bloody wound. Since it contains no nerves, it spares us intolerable pain from the interaction of our bodies with the environment. It is in the epidermis that callouses and blisters are built. These, too, are designed to protect the other layer of skin, the dermis (true skin, as it is known), and the subdermis, the active layer of tissue beneath the dermis.

But the epidermis is more than armor. It includes hair follicles, sweat glands, nails, and sebaceous glands. The activity or inactivity of the sebaceous glands is important in the skin's aging process because they produce sebum, a natural skin cream. Sebum contains waxes and fatty acids that destroy or inhibit the growth of germs on the skin. Found all over the body except in the palms, soles of the feet, and nails, sebaceous glands are particularly common in the face. Young healthy skin contains a greater number of active sebaceous glands than appear in older skin. The epitome of that is the adolescent boy suffering an acne attack. The glands are so plentiful and are functioning so well that they trap dirt and bacteria. If the face is not washed frequently—several times a day—the debris promptly forms a blackhead or whitehead.

Skin health and vitality depends in part upon healthy sebaceous glands and other epidermis cells. And the epidermis depends for its very existence on the layer below it, the dermis, a jellylike substance through which run the nerves, blood vessels, roots of the sweat and sebaceous glands, and a few random tissue fibers. Actually the dermis is called the "true skin" because it is the only living skin tissue. From it spring all the glands and cells of the epidermis. Our finger- and toenails, even the hair on our heads and bodies, are the progeny of the dermal cells.

The basic requirement of all body tissue is the same: adequate nutrition. The dermal cells are no exception. In fact, they are so sensitive to nutritional deficiencies that, particularly in the days when doctors did not have sophisticated diagnostic equipment, physicians relied extensively on the condition of the hair and the skin to determine nutritional and health status. A shortage of protein, the B vitamins, and several trace minerals are among the deficiencies which produce prompt adverse changes in the skin and hair.

Drs. Papa and Kligman wondered if there might not be another nutrient essential to healthy skin, one produced by the body itself—testosterone. The idea was not at all farfetched. Extensive studies had already shown that female hormones—estrogens—had some effect in keeping women's skin firm and healthy. But in the days preceding the nineteen sixties, men had been taught to frown upon any but the most basic concern for appearances. A man's wardrobe properly consisted of grays, dark blues, blacks, and browns. Loudness was fashionable only in ties, and beyond that frills and "silly" attempts at anything colorful, young, or strutting were derisively scorned as obviously effeminate.

As part of what *Look* magazine labeled the "Youthquake" of the nineteen sixties, males awakened to their own potential for attractiveness. In the backwash of the women's equality movement, men, particularly young ones, found a great deal of pleasure in wearing the latest men's fashions, the brightest colors, and the most sensuous fabrics. Older men started admitting that they did not like looking older after all, and there was nothing particularly silly or effeminate in doing what might be done to take a few years off their faces.

It was in that atmosphere that Papa and Kligman pursued their research. If estrogens had worked for women, perhaps testosterone would do the same for men. Thus they were led to the armpits of fourteen elderly men.

The preliminary findings were typical. The skin was drier, had less odor, and considerably fewer hairs than in younger men. Said the researchers, "The hair that is present is generally thin, wispy, and depigmented. Our qualitative studies show that sweating is considerably diminished, attributable, at least in part, to fewer functioning glands." Most sweat glands simply dry up like old dehydrated fruit.

Each of the volunteers was given a testosterone-containing ointment and instructed to rub it into the armpit every day for a full year. For comparison purposes the researchers selected three additional groups of men and tested three other ointments. One contained progesterone, another estrogen (both female hormones), and a third pregnenolone, a precursor to both male and female hormones.

According to Papa and Kligman, the skin of aging underarms is made up of fewer cell layers than that of younger men. The ridges are shallower, the cells irregular in size and shape. Instead of a network of well-shaped, healthy-looking cells found in young men, those of the aged seem to be separating from each other and deteriorating.

The elastic fiber, which in youth keeps the skin tight and rubbery, grows coarse with age and loses its springiness.

Say the researchers, "In extreme old age, cell depletion is a characteristic and obvious feature; the dermis seems lifeless . . . old skin appeared, in total, much like a neglected garden. The soil was dry and sandy, the plants withered and sparse. We were extremely skeptical that such skin could be importantly influenced, either for better or for worse."

Thus the researchers themselves were surprised to discover that the skin and the cells that composed it grew more youthful with testosterone. The cells became plump and more regular in size and shape, and, when tested for their reaction to enzymes, actually began to function in a more youthful manner than they had. The underarms began to exude more sweat and more odor. Now a perspiring and odorous armpit may not seem a positive achievement offhand, but at least in this case it was proof that cells which had shriveled and stopped functioning because of age were more youthful and active again.

Estrogens produced no results. According to the researchers, "The order of effectiveness of the steroids which bring about a partial reversal of the aging changes is testosterone, progesterone, and pregnenolone. Testosterone is far and away the most potent. Its effects are also the most consistent."

More than a quarter of a century ago Henry Turner, MD, wrote, in *Clinical Use of Testosterone*,

> Testosterone improves the nutrition of the skin of elderly, androgen-deficient subjects, who have pruritus and atrophy; and in some cases it benefits senile eczema. This may be regarded as an androgenic deficiency state, a complication of adult hypogonadism or the male climacteric. More basically, androgens affect the pigmentation, vascularity, and hair growth in the skin at all ages. The effect consists of improved oxygenation, probably a blood-vessel effect. . . .

Since Turner's writing, no findings have discounted his speculations. The fact that testosterone is essential in creating red blood cells which transport oxygen to the skin suggests that the hormone may indeed increase oxygenation of the skin cells. But more current research shows additional effects the androgen produces in the skin.

One has to do with the sebaceous glands mentioned earlier. Testosterone is not only involved in, but is primarily responsible for, sebaceous gland activity. One way that has been proven is by studying the sebum production in a group of elderly men castrated for medical reasons. In each case by the second month after the operation, a significant decrease in sebum secretions developed.

Even in women it seems that androgens, primarily testosterone secreted by the ovaries, have the major responsibility in stimulating sebaceous glands.

The sebaceous cells are certainly crucial to a healthy skin, but they do not explain all the observations made by Papa and Kligman. Nor does Turner's oxygenation theory. Neither alone would cause the cells to regain their original size and shape. That is accomplished through yet another phenomenon. Animal studies show that testosterone increases the skin's hyaluronate content. Hyaluronate increases the skin's permeability. It permits water molecules to enter the cells and swell them back to their youthful size and shape.

Dermatologist Dr. E.A. Davidson writes, in *Advances in Biology of Skin Aging*, Vol. 6 (edited by Montagna), "The result of the marked increased hyaluronate deposition in the skin is to increase the hydration level in the skin and to apparently reverse the time-dependent changes which have occurred in the composition of the skin polysaccharides. Thus the physiological picture of the skin of a testosterone-treated animal is that exhibited by an animal of younger chronological age."

The armpit study by Papa and Kligman left no doubt that topical, or surface, applications of testosterone can arrest and reverse skin aging. But the researchers made another discovery, too: Testosterone also affects body hair growth. At the beginning of the study the elderly volunteers had fewer underarm hairs, and those they had were thin, wispy, and depigmented (without color). Yet, following three or four months of daily hormone application, thirteen of the fourteen men showed what the investigators called a "striking increase in hair growth." Not only were there more hairs at a time in life when there would normally have been fewer, but the hairs were thicker and youthful in appearance.

Actually, the effect of testosterone—and all the androgens, in fact—on body hair growth has been well recognized for many years, and today the androgens are often prescribed for body hair when desired. Last year a twenty-four-year-old lead singer with a well-known rock group flew from his home in Chicago to New York City to visit dermatologist Norman Orentreich, MD. The young man had a rather common complaint, yet one that was troubling him sufficiently to warrant the trip to one of the nation's leading specialists.

"I'm a sex symbol, see?" he explained. "I gotta look tough, make 'em salivate a little. That's the game. You know, tight pants, bulging crotch, shirt open to the waist." He grimaced, disgusted. "Thing is, my chest's about as sexy as a marble. There ain't one hair growing on it!"

Orentreich injected small doses of testosterone in several areas beneath the skin of the chest. He also gave his patient a testosterone-containing lotion and instructed him to rub some of it into the skin once each day.

The young singer returned two months later for additional injections and more lotion. After another sixty days he made a third visit. It was his last, and to that appointment he wore a new custom-made shirt with plunging neckline. Like a peacock with its tail spread, the singer proudly sported a chest of luxuriant hair.

Such a feat is not in the least unusual. Thousands of young men each year seek out dermatologists to give their sluggish hair development a boost. Usually they suffer no defects whatever, except impatience. Their testes function normally and would eventually produce sufficient androgens to bring about the desired hair growth. But nature works at its own pace, and often neither rock singers nor others choose to wait.

Puzzling though it may seem, hair is closely related in its origin to finger- and toenails. All three are formed by collections of specialized epidermal cells. Hair begins growing from an indentation in the skin called a follicle. There, as Reginald T. Braim, MD, explains in his book, *Skin Diseases*, the base of a hair strand is formed by

> collections of specialized epidermal cells arranged as a cone, and these cells go through the changes of producing horny material just

> like the other epidermal cells. The hairs are built up from round, flat horny cells like little carved tiles around the central core of less organized material called the medulla of the hair. Pigment is deposited into these cells, and this accounts for the blond or brunet, according to the amount of dark pigment the hair contains. As the cylindrical shaft is formed, it is pushed upwards and runs between sheets of cells partly formed from the hair root and partly from the walls of the hair bulb or follicle which supports the hair in its progress from the root up to the skin surface.

When the hair is finally made, it is simply a pile of dead horny skin cells. Yet physicians can tell a great deal about the body's health by examining a strand of hair.

Normally hair cells contain a great many nutrients essential to the entire body. For example, each strand is made up of about 97 percent protein and 3 percent essential minerals and ash. The nutrients and oxygen are carried to the hair cells by an extensive network of blood vessels surrounding the follicles. By analyzing hair, physicians can determine with great accuracy the degree of mineral deficiency or imbalance, and thus can often prevent serious deficiency crises.

This information is important for some obvious reasons. One is that if the diet is deficient in essential nutrients, body hair may be sparse, brittle, or even virtually nonexistent. Certainly testosterone can no more build hair under such circumstances than nails can build a house. But such an extreme nutritional deficiency is probably rare. More common, particularly in older men, is progressive circulatory deficiency. If because of clogged capillaries, lower heart rate, and decreasing blood pressure, fewer nutrients and oxygen reach the hair follicles, decreasing hair growth must result. Thus hair growth requires adequate nutrition and physical condition.

Not all hair is the same, of course, not even on the same body. A person may have thick, flowing hair on his head; short, straight underarm hair; kinky and bristly pubic hair; and soft down on his arms. And the hair on his eyebrows may match none of the rest. One reason for these differences is that the follicles themselves vary in their structure and chemical requirements. The most obvious, and unfortunate, example is that follicles in most areas of both male and female bodies require androgens before they can produce hair cells. Yet most authorities agree that testosterone actually *prevents* follicles in the scalp from producing hair. Women treated with testosterone for various ailments such as breast cancer frequently develop a male-type baldness, and eunuchs and other men with very low testosterone levels never grow bald. The more heavily androgenized a man, the more likely his chances of baldness.

Of course nothing about the body's endocrine system is cut and dry; the relationship between androgens and baldness is no exception. A couple of studies have produced the startling finding that testosterone applications to the scalp have actually stimulated new hair growth in 75 percent of previously inactive follicles. But those results are opposed not only to the simple observation that highly masculinized middle-aged men frequently become bald, but also to laboratory findings of many studies.

Also, there seems to be an as yet unknown pituitary secretion that plays a part in body hair growth. So do the 17-ketosteroids from the adrenals, and they may stimulate hair growth on the scalp, too. Still, the primary stimulant to hair growth on the body, and lack of it on the scalp, is testosterone.

Thus one might expect men to display their bald pates as a proud hallmark of masculinity. That would be at least as appropriate as pride in bulging chests and biceps, but that is not likely to happen. Madison Avenue has too many men's hair products to sell to allow baldness to become part of the American way of life. We will continue to be sold the youth image. Men will be persuaded that baldness is not only somehow shameful, but a sign of lost sexuality. In the interest of unloading continued tons of hair sprays, lotions, shampoos, wigs, and such, the wavy-haired Latin lover will remain the ideal, and by implication the bald man will be considered undesirable.

Since things are not likely to change on Madison Avenue, the bald man has at least two quite obvious alternatives. He can stay bald, or he can buy himself some hair—transplant or wig. At this stage of endocrinology hormones cannot help.

12

Dimensions—Facts and Fancies

If there exists an outstanding all-American sexual neurosis, it has to do with penis size. Says James S. Glenn, MD, of Duke University School of Medicine, "It can be safely said that the adult male population suffers an almost universal anxiety in regard to penile size. The family physician and the urologist are often queried in this regard, and patients frequently express the feeling that they possess genitalia of inadequate or less than normal size." *Microphallneurosis,* as Dr. Glenn calls it, has become as basic to the American way of life as baseball and hot dogs.

That is not to say that microphallneurosis is unique to this culture or this age. In fact, evidence from many ancient civilizations, including India and Pompeii, shows that phallic dimensions were of great interest—so much so that artists and sculptors frequently enhanced the male genitalia to ludicrous proportions.

From those days to these, myriad formulas for phallic enlargement have been propounded and diligently used by those imagining themselves poorly endowed.

Shaykh Nefzawi, undoubtedly recognizing the universal obsession with phallic dimensions even in sixteenth-century Arabia, included instructions in *The Perfumed Garden* for enlarging the penis. Here is some of Nefzawi's interesting advice:

> A man, therefore, with a small member, who wants to make it grand or fortify it for the coitus, must rub it before copulation with tepid water, until it gets red and extended by the blood flowing into it, in consequence of the heat; he must then annoint it with a mixture of honey and ginger, rubbing it in sedulously. Then let him join the woman; he will procure for her such pleasure that she objects to him getting off her again.
>
> Another remedy consists in a compound made of a moderate quantity of pepper, lavender, galanga, and musk, reduced to powder, sifted, and mixed up with honey and preserved ginger. The member, after having been first washed in warm water, is then vigorously rubbed with the mixture; it will then grow large and brawny, and afford to the woman a marvelous feeling of voluptuousness.
>
> A third remedy is the following: Wash the member in warm water until it becomes red, and enters into erection. Then take a piece of soft leather, upon which spread hot pitch, and envelop the member with it. It will not be long before the member raises its head, trembling with passion.
>
> A fourth remedy is based upon the use made of leeches, but only of such that live in water. You put as many of them into a bottle as can be got in, and fill it up with oil. Then expose the bottle to the sun, until the heat of the same has effected a complete mixture. With the fluid thus obtained the member is to be rubbed several consecutive days, and it will, by being thus treated, become of a good size and of full dimensions.
>
> For another procedure I will here note the use of an ass' member. Procure one and boil it, with onions and a large quantity of corn. With this dish feed fowls, which you eat afterwards.
>
> Another way is to brew leeches with oil and rub the verge (penis) with this ointment; or the leeches may be put into a bottle, and buried in a warm dunghill until they are dissolved and form a sort of liniment, which is used for repeatedly annointing the member. The member is certain to greatly benefit by this.

Nefzawi assures his readers, "The efficacy of all these remedies is well-known, and I have tested them." To offset any doubts that we might still harbor, he tells the story of Abbés, whose member was very small. Abbés seemed to have been born under a falling star, for his problem was compounded by a corpulent wife. His deficiency and her excess made copulation impossible. What's more, Abbés depended on her fortune for his living expenses, since she was wealthy and he poor. But as his wife's sexual tension grew more and more frustrating month after month, she refused him a dime, and told all her girlfriends what a failure he was.

Abbés finally visited a sage and confessed his problem. The wise man declared, "If you had a fine member, her fortune would be yours. Do you not know that women's religion is in their vulvas? But I will prescribe you a remedy which will do away with your troubles."

We are not told precisely what the formula included. No doubt it was one of the recipes Nefzawi himself prescribed. Of course it had the effect of making Abbés' member long and thick. When his wife saw it, she was stunned with joy.

"But it was still better when he made her feel in the matter of enjoyment quite another thing than she had been accustomed to experience," Nefzawi tells us. "He began in fact to work her with his tool in quite a remarkable manner, to such a point that she trembled and sighed and sobbed and cried out during the operation." As might be expected, she gleefully turned over to Abbés her entire fortune and devoted herself to him happily ever after.

Nefzawi's procedures, peculiar though they were, are no more fanciful than some actually practiced by so-called therapists even today. One who made headlines not long ago is Robert Peterson of the New Life Clinic of Fort Myers, Florida. Before being exposed and indicted on twenty counts, Peterson proclaimed that he frequently added length and circumference to a man's penis through the following process:

An adult ram is suspended from the ceiling by its hind legs. An assistant slashes the jugular vein and the animal bleeds to death.

The cadaver is pushed through a sliding window into a second room. There Peterson removes the testicles and hands them to assistants in a third room. These people grind the organs, mixing them with the sex glands taken from a sheep fetus. Later, the substance is injected into the man seeking an enlarged phallus.

A new approach to penile enlargement in recent years is the plastic suction pump sold by mail and in adult bookstores and novelty shops. The penis is inserted into the device and the air withdrawn, producing a vacuum which causes the penis to enlarge. Fluid rushes into the penis and does temporarily swell the cells of the organ, so that for a short time—a few hours—the user has his wish, a noticeably enlarged penis. No harmful effects from using the gadget have been reported, and it may serve as a pleasant amusement. But it certainly does not produce permanently enlarged sex organs.

The universality of microphallneurosis becomes all the more curious when it is recognized that penile dimensions are more or less standard. Certainly there are extremes. Some men are born with no external genitalia at all. And although many wild claims have been made for maximum sizes—up to 22 inches—the more reliable studies agree on about 13¾ inches. Average length, according to Masters and Johnson and others, is from 4½ to 8 inches during full erection, with the great majority being 5¾ to 6 inches long. Only about one man in a hundred will have an organ either smaller or larger than average. It must be remembered that a penis is never too small unless, as in the case of Nefzawi's Abbés, it is incapable of penetration. Often the opposite is true, in fact—the larger the penis, the less functional it may be. For example, sex therapists and gynecologists are far more familiar with female complaints of pain created by large male organs than by expressions of dissatisfaction with inadequate penetration.

Frequently, extended oral intercourse is impossible for the woman whose partner has a larger than average phallus. Sexual activity is therefore limited to the more routine genital-to-genital contact and masturbation. And, although apparently no formal study has ever been conducted to prove it, a widely held opinion is that particularly large penises do not attain the degree of rigidity in erection that is achieved by smaller ones. All in all, it is probably the man with the normal size penis rather than the Ringling Brothers extravaganza who is most fortunate.

For the man who is truly microphallic, testosterone can help *sometimes.* More than a decade ago a thirty-eight-year-old man came to the Baltimore office of Dr. Virginia Huffer complaining of physical weakness. At six feet one inch in height and 179 pounds he did not *look* weak, just very youthful. His face was beardless, puffy, and pale; his voice high-pitched. At first the doctor guessed he was a teenager.

Twenty-two years earlier he had consulted a physician because he had failed to develop sexually as other sixteen-year-old males had. The doctor assured him nothing could be done, and on that professional advice the man, throughout his twenties and thirties, endured physical weakness and embarrassment because of his immature appearance and was deprived of all sexual desire and activity.

A series of tests showed that the man's pituitary was not secreting thyroid and gonad-stimulating hormones. For four months Dr. Huffer prescribed thyroid hormones only, and the patient's physical endurance increased. Then, at his request, she administered testosterone injections. The most significant change, in Huffer's words: "Small doses of testosterone preparation during the next year resulted in significant enlargement of his phallus. . . ."

He became a sexual being. During treatment he was aware of three or four erections nightly. He began masturbating several times weekly. Erotic fantasies involving girls he knew began to occupy his thoughts. Even at age thirty-eight testosterone had helped this person along the road to normal manhood.

An interesting epilogue to this story: The patient responded to his own erotic impulses with anxiety and depression. He said he felt he was "too old" to start thinking about sex, and he could not develop the courage to pursue a girl, date her, attempt to make love to her, and so forth. He abruptly discontinued all therapy, but eventually returned for thyroid hormones, specifying that he was not interested in testosterone.

To avoid emotional difficulties like those, Herbert Kupperman, MD, recommends that determining the degree of genital development be part of any routine adolescent physical examination. "If sex hormone therapy is needed, it should be given early—as close as possible to the time when the body itself would be producing the hormones," he says. "The alternative—

placing a thirty- or forty-year-old man into an adolescent sexual development phase—creates an emotional trauma that could be overwhelming."

There is another good reason for treating the adolescent rather than the adult: In some cases a small penis cannot be made to grow larger in adulthood. Often tests show that a young man is endocrinologically normal, i.e., he is producing sufficient testosterone to meet his needs. His phallus, while significantly smaller than those of other boys his age, is about the same size as other men in his family, and that indicates that he is genetically programmed to have small sex organs.

Many physicians today would conclude that this boy could not be helped. If a young man has already reached his genetic potential, no amount of testosterone can help him do more.

But some endocrinologists specializing in precisely this problem say these young men can indeed be helped. They argue that rarely if ever do normal people reach their maximum genetic capacity. As we mentioned earlier, we have the potential to produce denser bones, stronger muscles, sounder cardiovascular systems, perhaps even greater intelligence by varying environmental and nutritional factors. Those physical changes would be impossible if we started out at our maximum potential genetic size. The same is true of penile dimensions. Whether a penis is two inches or twelve inches, it is undoubtedly the product of its possessor's *normal* genetic expression, but not the maximum possible. By making available additional testosterone to these sex glands while they are in the growing stage, additional size can often be attained.

Says Dr. J. H. Vogelman of the Orentreich Foundation for the Advancement of Science, "The norm in sexual development is obviously less than the maximum possible genetic expression. For that reason I would guess that a significant proportion of the male population could increase penis size to some degree."

Dr. Kupperman has treated hundreds of cases of microphallus in otherwise normal young men. "If we can treat these young men in their adolescence, we can expect one hundred percent success," he says. "It is only after they have gone on to adulthood and their bodies have stopped growing that therapy becomes difficult. Not only do they face the normal adolescent/adult adjustment at an age when it is difficult to cope with such problems, but there is the possibility that their bodies will not respond as expected to the hormones. What's more, they have often already developed emotional problems resulting from their physical inadequacy."

One example of effective testosterone therapy is a young teenager who was so ashamed of his physical inadequacy that he dropped out of high school rather than be jeered in the locker room by his normally developed classmates. By age fifteen, he had made a more or less feminine identification and had developed a passive personality. One of his favorite pastimes was to bake pies for his mother.

Much as the woman enjoyed the pies, she was profoundly troubled by her son's lack of masculine characteristics. She sought Dr. Kupperman's help and he immediately began testosterone therapy. Within three months the boy underwent a physical and mental metamorphosis. His phallus enlarged, his voice deepened, he began growing body hair. In dealing with others he became more self-assertive. One matter in particular amused his mother—he refused to bake any more pies, explaining that she could do the baking from then on and he would do the eating.

Kupperman estimates that perhaps ten percent of preadolescent boys have small penises. That is no call for concern. About three fourths of them will develop normally. Of those who do not, the doctor must first conduct the standard tests we have already discussed to determine testosterone and pituitary gonadotrophin levels. He may find that all systems are functioning adequately and decide to give testosterone to press development from the young man's normal genetic size to its maximum potential. Or the physician may elect to give a pituitary gonad-stimulating hormone, pushing the testes to work harder and produce additional testosterone.

If the man is approaching twenty, the doctor may first want to learn whether or not he is still growing, for if growth has ceased, the hormone will do no good in a normal young man. An x-ray will show whether or not the epiphyses, or bone fragments in youthful skeletons, have fused with larger bones as they do in adults, signifying the completion of growth. If that has taken place, testosterone will be of little use.

In some men, however, this epiphyseal fusion never takes place because, unlike normal adolescents with small penises, these others are hypogonadal—they do not produce testosterone. It is testosterone which prompts the bone to fuse. As long as the bones stay immature, growth continues (often producing very tall, gangly men). If the man is hypogonadal, his penis can be stimulated to grow larger, regardless of his age.

But the point, once again, is that subnormal penis size is a rarity. Only *concern* about it is common. If what is needed is assurance, a tape measure can provide that for ninety-nine out of a hundred men. The measurement is taken from the upper side of the erect shaft, the end of the measure pressed firmly against the pubic hair at the abdomen. If you measure at least four and a half inches, relax and enjoy it. If not, see an endocrinologist.

13
Not Enough

About a hundred fifty miles west of Santo Domingo in the Dominican Republic there is a small, isolated village called Salinas. About four thousand people live there. It is in almost every way a typical South American town and population.

One characteristic distinguishes it. Approximately one out of every ninety boys is born with undescended testes and a scrotum which lifts high into the abdomen, so that it appears to be female labia rather than the male genitalia. The penis is so small it is easily mistaken for a clitoris. The villagers cannot be blamed for assuming these infants are girls, and they are reared as such. The children themselves seem perfectly content with that.

Then at puberty something of a miracle takes place. The "girls" develop deeper voices. Their bodies grow strong and muscular. They do not develop breasts, and their "clitorises" enlarge to many times the previous size. That development is so profound that the townspeople actually call these youngsters *guevedocos*, meaning "penis at twelve years of age."

There are other changes, too. The scrotum enlarges and the testes descend into it. Male internal sex glands develop and begin producing sperm and prostatic fluid. Now the children have become boys, and, interestingly, they make a thoroughgoing masculine orientation.

Researchers from the Division of Endocrinology at Cornell

University's Medical College heard the story of the *guevedocos* and their curiosity was piqued. The mystery was compounded by reports from others that the children had every bit as much testosterone in their systems as other boys did. The researchers decided to investigate, but even before they boarded the plane for Santo Domingo, they had developed a theory. It centered on the fact that, while pure testosterone is needed by some of the body's cells, others cannot use it as it is secreted by the testes. It must first undergo a minor conversion to *dihydro*testosterone (DHT). Ordinarily the conversion occurs as a simple, natural process in testosterone utilization. Yet the researchers were almost certain the delayed sexual development of the *guevedocos* was caused by a breakdown in the testosterone/dihydrotestosterone conversion.

In Salinas the researchers first confirmed that testosterone levels were well within normal range. Then they checked for the dihydrotestosterone and found, as expected, that it was low—in some *guevedocos* it reached only one sixth of the normal level.

Tracing the cause of medical problems can often be like seeking Kafka's castle, an endless maze of wandering into blind alleys and dead ends. But at least one fact was clear to the investigators: If the conversion from testosterone to dihydrotestosterone did not take place, it was almost certainly because the essential enzyme to trigger it was absent. That enzyme has the jawbreaker name, delta 4 steroid 5 alpha (or beta) reductase. The enzyme performs the conversion in the liver and also in "target cells," those that need the dihydrotestosterone.

The *guevedocos* are a good example of what happens when insufficient testosterone (in one form or another) reaches the target cells of certain male sex glands. The body fails to masculinize normally, to break away entirely from its basic congenital femaleness. The *guevedocos* illustrate another point, too: Often what appears to be a simple testosterone deficiency is much more complex, sometimes involving enzymes, other hormones, hormone-binding globulins, target organ insensitivity, and such. The matter grows very complex, and there is no need to discuss here in great detail such exotic problems as the *guevedocos* of Salinas. Far more important are the *common* causes of feminization in men.

Klinefelter's syndrome

Perhaps the most common feminizing disease is Klinefelter's syndrome. It affects one out of every four hundred males. The youth suffering Klinefelter's syndrome is usually dismissed as just a fat kid who cannot control his eating habits. In fact, he probably was never an overeater. Yet there is no denying the excess fat, particularly around the breasts and upper thighs. A roll of fat, different from the typical middle-aged potbelly, may gather in rings around the hips and stomach. Even if he is grossly underweight, he is not able to shed the gynecomastia, or breast development, and fat accumulation on the thighs. The penis may be normal, but the testes are noticeably small—less than half the expected size.

His doctor will take blood and urine samples, send them to a laboratory, and thus learn the pituitary is sending high levels of gonadotrophin to the testes. But the testes are not responding. A semen sample will show complete absence of sperm. A biopsy, or sample of testicular tissue, must be taken to confirm the Klinefelter's syndrome diagnosis. Under a microscope the doctor will recognize that the interstitial cells and seminiferous tubules are greatly reduced in number and are deformed.

The damage to the testes is an irony: It is caused by a lack of the testosterone the testes themselves produce. The cells which make up the tubules of the testes are "androgen insensitive"; because of a genetic error, they cannot absorb the testosterone they need, like all sex organs. The undeveloped tubules fail to produce the hormone, and the problem is compounded.

Since the ailment is genetic, it cannot be cured, but it can be treated by testosterone replacement therapy. No matter at what age testosterone treatment begins, the body will take on a more masculine appearance and sexual capacity will increase.

Eunuchoidism

Another testosterone deficiency disease is eunuchoidism. The victim has overall a more feminine body than the Klinefelter's patient. He has narrow shoulders, wide hips, and long arms. Like his counterpart, he may develop femalelike breasts. His penis will either be very small or microphallic (almost nonexistent), and there will be little or no prostatic development.

Laboratory tests may show findings similar to those of Klinefelter's syndrome, except that the testicular biopsy will reveal not only deformity but complete destruction of the interstitial cells. The eunuchoid man can be dramatically helped by testosterone therapy, for he does not suffer androgen insensitivity in sex tissue cells, but a frank testosterone deficiency.

On occasion it is not the testes themselves which malfunction but the pituitary. If the pituitary does not produce gonad-stimulating hormones, the testes will not produce testosterone. Lab tests can quickly determine that by analyzing blood and urine for pituitary gonadotrophins. Preferred treatment, particularly in adolescence, is human chorionic gonadotrophin (HCG), a hormone derived from the urine of pregnant women. It stimulates the testes to function normally, acting as a substitute for the pituitary gonadotrophins.

Cryptorchidism

Another testosterone deficiency problem is cryptorchidism. Three percent of all full-term male infants and 21 percent of premature ones are born with one or both testicles undescended. About 80 percent of the time the testes will descend normally into the scrotum during the first year of life. When they do not, medical intervention is essential.

Sometimes the doctor can manipulate the glands into place. When the cremasteric muscle contracts and thus holds the testicle in the abdomen, the physician can often relax the muscle through massage, and that may allow the testes to drop. Sometimes an experienced physician will simply ask the child to squat, and the testis will occasionally descend of its own accord. Human chorionic gonadotrophin, the hormone mentioned above, may also stimulate the testes to descend.

If those procedures fail, surgery is required, for an undescended testicle is a potentially dangerous problem. The testes are not capable of functioning adequately when exposed to the body's normal temperature of 98.6°F, so nature prepared the scrotum for their dwelling place. When the body is particularly warm, the scrotal skin actually expands, allowing the testes to drop several inches away from the body in order to maintain a lower temperature. And when the testes are exposed to cold water or air, the scrotum contracts, bringing them in closer contact with the warm body, but still far enough away to prevent overheating.

It is a very delicate mechanism, this process of regulating precisely the temperature to which the testes are exposed. And it is essential, for too much cold or heat—and the body temperature *is* too much—promptly kills sperm and prevents the seminiferous tubules from functioning. Chronic excess temperatures will actually destroy the tubules. The interstitial cells still function to produce testosterone, but may age much more rapidly than normal and ultimately cease hormone production. The body's heat can cause permanent damage to undescended testicles beginning as early as the fourth or fifth year of life.

Still more important, after age twenty undescended testicles are prone to become cancerous. Once again human chorionic gonadotrophin (HCG) is the preferred treatment. Hopefully that will bring about the conclusion of growth process in the developing testes so that they will descend as they should have at birth. If that fails, orchiopexy should be performed. This is an operation in which the surgeon physically attaches the testis to the scrotum so that it cannot contract again into the body.

The operation does not guarantee that cancer won't develop, however. Any man who has reached adolescence with an undescended testicle should have physical examinations at least twice a year, for the damage that could lead to cancer has already occurred.

Anorchism

Anorchism, the complete absence of testes, can be mistaken for cryptorchidism, although it is not as common. The scrotum, of course, is empty. The body characteristics are similar to those of a male with undescended testes. If human chorionic gonadotrophin does not lead to increased urinary estrogen and testosterone levels and an increasingly masculine body, anorchism is the likely diagnosis. There simply are no testes for the HCG to stimulate. The only solution is lifelong androgen replacement.

Infertility

Infertility is another problem sometimes related to testosterone deficiency. A normal male releases about 400 million live spermatozoa in an average ejaculation. If the seminal fluid contains less than 20 million sperm, he is considered probably infertile. Thousands of men seek help every year for this problem, but Hugh Lamensdorf, MD, summarized the state of treatment concisely in the May, 1975, issue of *Fertility and Sterility:*

> After complicated endocrine assays, testicular biopsies, and considerable expense, most patients are found to have no treatable disease. Because of these disappointing results, most physicians have abandoned complicated investigations and fall into the easy habit of using empiric medication with thyroid extracts, vitamin and mineral supplements, or low doses of testosterone, knowing all the while that they will not improve the patient's fertility.

Probably the most promising approach to infertility now available was recognized more than a quarter of a century ago by Dr. C. G. Heller, currently of the Division of Reproductive Physiology at the Pacific Northwest Research Foundation in Seattle. Yet even today few physicians are aware of Heller's research. It may be that most never got beyond the first half of Heller's findings, the seemingly negative fact that testosterone in large doses actually causes the seminiferous tubules of the testes, where the sperm are made, to degenerate. (It does the same to the interstitial cells which produce testosterone.) The hormone, by destroying the sperm-making equipment, seems to cause, not cure, infertility. Most doctors know that but are not familiar with the more significant aspect of Heller's report. Addressing the 1950 meeting of the American Society for the Study of Sterility, he went on to explain that once hormone doses are discontinued, new, healthy seminiferous tubules replace the original ones.

Immediately after Heller's report other researchers confirmed his findings, and for a while fertility doctors showed great enthusiasm for testosterone therapy. Then suddenly it lost favor. One reason was the discovery that only twenty men out of a hundred fathered a child after the new therapy. (Overlooked was the fact that *all* of these men had failed to respond to other approaches, and most likely *none* would have become fathers without Heller's treatment.)

The second criticism was more significant. On occasion the germinal epithelium did not regenerate and there was even less sperm production than before.

Yet some therapists continued to prescribe testosterone for infertility, assuming that the risk was merely to maintain the status quo, and the potential reward far outweighed that. One of these practitioners was Dr. Lamensdorf. He has been prescribing testosterone for the past twenty-two years with what he calls "a moderate degree of success." Specifically, of 145 men treated, 39 (27 percent) ultimately impregnated their wives. Some of them had produced virtually no sperm before the testosterone treatment. In others, the sperm had been unhealthy and showed little movement.

Three patients (two percent) suffered permanent seminiferous tubule damage.

In July, 1972, Heller himself, along with Mavis J. Rowley, reported in the professional journal, *Fertility and Sterility,* on 157 cases of infertility he had treated during the previous eighteen years. Each of the men and their wives had been attempting conception unsuccessfully for between two and sixteen years.

Each patient was committed to a full two-year program during which he was given sufficient testosterone as well as female hormones to eliminate totally all sperm production. Then the treatment was stopped, and within six months to two years, 110 of the treatment programs resulted in a statistically significant increase in sperm concentration. Of the remainder, thirteen led to a decrease, twenty-four produced no obvious change, and the remainder were not adequately followed up.

More than 40 percent of the men succeeded in impregnating

their wives as a result of treatment. Of those who failed, three divorced their wives before the treatment effect could be determined. One died. The wife of another underwent a hysterectomy. And eighty-three dropped out of the program before the observation period was complete. That is important, for most conceptions took place during the second year following the end of therapy, and of those, more than half occurred in the last six months of the second year. Many of the dropouts may have produced children.

More than half of these men who had been trying unsuccessfully to father offspring for up to sixteen years had two or more children within four years after the treatment program.

The most interesting aspect of the study concerns the thirteen men who, following treatment, showed a decrease in their sperm counts. Each recovered to an average of only 60 percent of their pretreatment levels. Yet ten of those thirteen had far fewer abnormal sperm than before, and following the therapy, even though their sperm levels were lower, five of them impregnated their wives.

Gynecomastia,

or abnormal breast development in males, is common. About 95 percent of boys entering puberty experience it to some degree. It is usually harmless, except psychologically, yet frequently unexplainable. Testosterone deficiency is certainly related to some cases—gynecomastia is often one of the side effects of subnormal testosterone production. But the breasts may enlarge when testosterone levels are normal because of high estrogen secretions. Even when both are normal, pituitary hormones can trigger gynecomastia.

Researcher J. W. Jull, PhD, after studying fifteen cases, pointed out the complexity of causes: "Three (of the fifteen cases) can be explained on the basis of abnormally low estrogen production, two cases were probably due to pubertal increases in pituitary activity, and five were consequent upon increased estrogen secretion. In the remaining five cases some other cause of increased breast growth must be sought."

The man experiencing excess breast development should undergo tests to determine the reason, even if he is not particularly concerned with his appearance. Gynecomastia might indicate an endocrine tumor, and an early diagnosis can be lifesaving.

Excess estrogens

Frequently testosterone deficiency problems are traceable to excess estrogens, alluded to earlier as the hormonal equivalent to the eternal battle of the sexes. Often testosterone secretion will be solidly within normal range, but estrogen production may be two or three times the expected.

That excess estrogen has many effects on the male body. One has to do with sex hormone binding globulin (SBG), the proteins mentioned in Chapter 8 (Cycles and Variations), which are produced in the liver and bind with sex hormones in the blood. We have seen that while the hormones are bound with SBG, they cannot be utilized by the body. An excess of SBG causes a functional testosterone deficiency, whether or not adequate testosterone is being produced by the testes.

Both androgens and estrogens stimulate SBG production. That is one way the body maintains optimal blood hormone levels. But when excess estrogens are produced, more SBG is called for. That would not be much of a problem if SBG binded primarily with estrogens, but it does not. In fact, the reverse is true—SBG binds preferentially with testosterone, leaving the estrogens free to feminize the body.

In the normal male testosterone actually depresses SBG production, and in the normal woman estrogen stimulates it. Thus sex hormone binding globulin (SBG) helps maintain our sexual identity. In women it keeps testosterone levels low, and in men testosterone keeps SBG low so that masculinity can be asserted. Thus men produce about one half as much SBG as women do.

Probably the original defect which permits excess estrogen occurs in the interstitial cells of the testes, where about two thirds of male estrogen secretions are produced. For reasons not yet known some men are hypersecretors of estrogen. The normal man produces about seventy-five times as much *free* testosterone as does a woman, but as the ratio between testosterone and estrogen decreases, so do masculine characteristics.

But the body is no slipshod, thrown-together, assembly-line hunk of junk. It has been modified and perfected through millions of years, and one of the great marvels of its development is its series of checks and balances. Figuratively speaking, nature is eager that men and women remain biologically distinct. Thus, should a set of testes produce too much estrogen—and considering the precarious embryonic development of the male, there is every reason to suspect that it might—nature has developed a fail-safe method of preserving manhood. One of the liver's many jobs is to detoxify excess estrogens.

According to esteemed endocrinologist Mortimer Lipsett, any disease or malfunction of the liver can affect the body's hormone balance. Perhaps that may explain the general observation that chronic excess drinkers and alcoholics seem to have lower sex drives than does the general male population. Long before cirrhosis of the liver develops, alcohol causes abnormal changes in liver cells.

Another result of liver disease: higher blood SBG levels. Several studies show that. For example, Dr. David Anderson of the Medical Professorial Unit of St. Bartholomew's Hospital, London, found that twenty-five men with chronic liver disease, eight of them alcoholic cirrhotics, had significantly higher than normal sex hormone binding globulin levels. Anderson theorizes that the hypogonadism and gynecomastia which are seen especially in alcoholic cirrhotics develop for two reasons—the increased SBG excessively binds testosterone, and estrogens are not detoxified.

These are merely the more common of numerous reasons a man may fail to develop to his full masculine potential. Adrenal glands that produce inadequate levels of 17-ketosteroid precursors will encourage decreased masculinity. So will a diseased hypothalamus or pituitary. Any ailments that interfere with blood circulation can reduce the efficient functioning of the entire hypothalamic-pituitary-gonadal axis.

And even these problems are but the tip of the iceberg, the fraction we know about. Still eluding the endocrinologist's curiosity are the awesome and perhaps very basic secrets of hormone interactions—the subtleties of their influences. New hormones are being discovered continually, and important new findings on hormonal function are even more frequent.

Continuing endocrinologic research and nothing else will ultimately uncover the specific causes of sexual subdevelopment among men. When that day comes, treatment will be available from conception through adulthood to assure normal development for those men who desire it. Until then we will go on treating the symptoms, throwing water on fires that should never have started in the first place.

14
Sex Man to Man

Shortly after testosterone was isolated and synthesized in the nineteen thirties, some researchers hypothesized that a deficiency of the hormone in some men was the primary cause of homosexuality, transvestism (playacting an opposite sex role, including cross-dressing), and transsexualism (actually identifying psychologically with and desiring to be a member of the opposite sex). Since urine analysis had been developed to indicate testosterone production levels, the necessary research seemed simple. Several investigators set out to determine the hormonal difference between homosexuals and heterosexuals.

Unfortunately for the researchers, the results were almost as varied as the number of studies. No doubt that was partly because the only testosterone measuring method available then was a clumsy biological test, tedious, prolonged, and not always accurate. It was not until recently that a far superior method of determining blood testosterone levels was developed, and that gave rise to a new battery of studies intended to determine the hormone/homosexual link.

One investigation that received widespread attention was by Dr. Robert C. Kolodny and his associates at the famed Reproductive Biology Research Foundation at the Washington University School of Medicine in St. Louis. Kolodny used for his study thirty homosexual college students. But from the outset he recognized that some significant distinctions among homosexuals would be necessary. For example, a happily married heterosexual man who occasionally has sex with a male friend is not homosexual in the same sense as the man who has four or five male lovers a week and is not interested in heterosexual contact. Including both groups in a study of homosexuality would not present useful findings. Kolodny decided to rely on a standard scale of degree of hetero/homosexuality devised years ago by pioneer sex researcher Alfred Kinsey.

Kinsey classified all men according to one of six categories. Category 1 men are exclusively heterosexual, Category 6 exclusively homosexual. According to the Kinsey scale, the men in Category 3 would be the true bisexuals—those who are more or less equally active sexually with men and women and who enjoy both relationships and have no preferences. Kolodny's homosexuals were Kinsey-rated 5 and 6 only.

Examining a control group of exclusively heterosexual college men, Kolodny found blood testosterone levels of a 689-billionth of a gram for 100 cubic centimeters of blood. He compared that with the exclusive homosexuals and found their testosterone levels reduced by 60 percent. Men who were predominantly homosexual but who had incidental heterosexual experiences had hormone levels about 54 percent of the heterosexual average.

Kolodny also checked sperm production levels. His volunteers were asked to postpone all ejaculations for seventy-two hours and then to masturbate. Analysis of the semen samples showed that nine of the fifteen men in Kinsey's Categories 5 and 6 had below normal sperm counts. Four had no sperm at all, and half of the others produced sperm with impaired motility.

More recently another study published in the *Journal of Sex Research* involved a variety of sex deviates. (Unfortunately the word "deviate" has come to assume negative connotations. In usage here it defines one whose practices differ, or deviate, from the majority.) In addition to the 79 "normal" men, L. Starka and colleagues tested 17 male transsexuals, 3 transvestites, 18 male homosexuals with feminine disposition, and 3 male homosexuals who appeared masculine. Concluded the authors, "When the number of values lower than that in the normal range is compared in the groups of psychosexual deviates and in normal men, a significant depression of circulating testosterone can be demonstrated."

Soon after the Kolodny and Starká studies were published, the critics began pointing out their weaknesses. One man in Kolodny's group, a Category 3 true bisexual, had higher testosterone levels than any of the 689 control heterosexuals. Does the exception prove the rule or disprove it? Starká's feminine-type homosexuals have higher testosterone levels than do the masculine type. And his transsexuals, who are psychosexually thoroughgoing females, have higher levels than transvestites (who are frequently *not* homosexual in their partner preferences, but lead happy, well-adjusted sex lives and simply prefer to dress in women's clothes). The transsexuals had higher testosterone levels than even the masculine homosexuals. What's more, Starká tells us that among the eighteen feminine homosexuals two were actually in the upper normal limits and eight were in average normal limits of blood testosterone. None of these feminine men had extremely low testosterone levels.

Predictably, new studies were undertaken to determine the truth. This time Peter Doerer, MD, and his colleagues at the Max Planck Institute for Psychiatry in Munich investigated testosterone blood levels of thirty-two homosexuals. Concluded Dr. Doerer, "It is obvious that the homosexual group did not differ from the control group, and there is no relationship between the plasma testosterone levels and the Kinsey (homo/heterosexuality) ratings."

Unlike Kolodny he found no significant difference in sperm production or fertility levels. Dr. Doerer also checked the blood levels of a particular estrogen—estradiol. He found, "The median of the homosexual group is 27 percent higher than that of the control group."

Then, in 1974, Gary A. Parks of the New York Hospital—Cornell Medical Center in New York City, along with other researchers, published a study which discounted all those that had gone before. He showed, as we have already seen in Chapter 8, that extreme cyclic variations occur by the moment as well as by hours, days, and weeks in testosterone production. Further, wide variations exist among men in normal levels of production and efficiency of utilization. Dr. Parks pointed out that no previous studies had taken these factors into account.

Parks did his own investigation involving twelve boys between the ages of fifteen and nineteen. Half were homosexual and half heterosexual. He took blood samples for twenty-eight consecutive days and found that, although there were great day-to-day variations in hormone levels, when these were averaged out, no significant differences existed.

It was only a matter of time before a study would come along with findings to complete the cycle. It was published in the *American Journal of Psychiatry* in January, 1974, and was the work of H. Keith Brodie, MD, and co-workers. It was as sophisticated a testing method as Parks used. For one thing, all nineteen homosexuals were Kinsey Group 6 exclusively. The controls were exclusively heterosexual, with no history at all of homosexual activity.

The blood samples were taken at eight o'clock every other morning for a week and carefully analyzed. Brodie and his assistants concluded that the plasma testosterone level of the *heterosexual* subjects "was significantly lower than the mean plasma testosterone level for the homosexual men."

Now homosexuals had more testosterone than heterosexuals! The extremes within the range of levels were approximately the same—both lowest and highest levels were found in the heterosexuals.

Thus everyone was free to answer the homosexual/hormone question any way he wished and could find scientific research to support his position. The confusion was nothing new to researchers investigating the etiology of homosexuality. Before the biochemical approach gained popularity, they had been struggling with a grand array of theories from psychiatry, psychotherapy, and psychoanalysis. The dominant mother and passive, aloof father had gained wide attention. Overly protective and possessive mothers were considered at fault. One psychologist proposed that boys reared in the presence of an older *sister* had tendencies toward sexual repugnance and avoided heterosexual relationships. Yet the same year that study was reported, Dr. John Money of Johns Hopkins University's department of medicine wrote in the *Psychological Bulletin* (1970) that he had found what seemed to be a tendency for homosexual men to have more brothers than expected, and in these families there is a *shortage* of sisters.

The latest evidence denies any environmental causes of homosexuality. Dr. Bernard Zuger, clinical psychiatrist at New York University School of Medicine, reported a study in the February, 1970, issue of the *American Journal of Psychiatry,* demonstrating that twenty-five persistently effeminate young boys were carefully investigated, and Zuger determined that family histories were in no way significantly different from that of normal youngsters. On the whole, mothers were not particularly dominant or suffocating. The fathers were clearly the leaders of the household and showed a typical amount of affection and attention for their sons. Zuger's conclusion: Effeminate behavior "is inherent in the boys themselves."

The trouble with all this research, however, is the apparently persistent effort to explain with a single answer the reasons a man may become homosexual. We would not dream of doing that with other behavioral traits. For example, we might say that a man is ambitious in business because he learned to behave that way through a father's example. On the other hand, his father may have been inordinately lazy and his family oppressed with poverty; and in violent rejection of that he determined to be a financial success. Perhaps his adrenal glands are hyperactive, the hormones they secrete stimulating him to work day and night. Or he may be suffering a pituitary tumor, and that deadly growth could be secreting excess hormones which whip him on to success.

No therapist today would seriously consider that all depression is caused by a single factor. We know it results from feelings of unworthiness, self-doubt, loss, illness, nutritional deficiency, and a host of biochemical imbalances.

Yet research involving homosexuality still frequently persists in the pursuit of the single cause. As long as studies are undertaken from that perspective, results will continue to be conflicting and contradictory.

What *has* become obvious from the research conducted thus far is that some homosexuals—and only some—are biologically and genetically programmed in that direction even before birth. Extensive interviews with homosexuals reveal that, even when some of these men were very young, they recalled having a strong sexual attraction to other boys, and also to adult men. While attraction to boys and men was not unheard of among those who grew up to be heterosexuals, it was far less frequent. Yet both groups came from the same type of environment, suggesting that early sexual interests were in some way inherent in the children.

From animal research laboratories comes more hard-nosed scientific evidence. Researchers at the University of Kansas showed that if testosterone was not made available to the brain of a rat at a crucial point in its early development, the rat would develop the psychosexual characteristics of a female, whether or not the body was male. Alternately, if testosterone was supplied to the brain, the rodent would become psychosexually male, regardless of its body sex.

Rats are born, in a sense, prematurely, and so the critical period of the brain's sexual differentiation is up to four days following birth. But essentially the same effect has been demonstrated in guinea pigs and monkeys, and in these cases of longer-gestating animals, the brain's sexual orientation occurs before birth. Man, with a still longer gestation period, would presumably undergo psychosexual orientation during the early fetal stage.

The precise process whereby the brain is sexually differentiated is spelled out by Dr. Money in the *Psychological Bulletin*:

> When radioactive-labeled male hormone is administered to the fetus either through the mother or directly, in the case of the rat which is born immature, its uptake can be traced to various organs, including cells in the hypothalamus. When the hormone is administered within the critical period, if the fetus is a genetic

female, the hypothalamic nuclei will be masculinized. These cells will never be able to release their neurohumoral messages to the pituitary in the cyclic fashion characteristic of the female.... Because other hypothalamic nuclei that regulate sexual behavior will have been affected by the male hormone, the animal's behavior will not conform to that of the normal female. Typically, the animal will be disoriented and disorganized in its sexual response, or will repulse the male.

While appearing to be a normal female, this animal will be uninterested in heterosexual activity. But what about the rat with a biologically male body? We know that the basic development of the fetus, including that of the rat, is female. Only testosterone can cause the fetus to evolve or mutate into a male. That process involves, first, the masculinization of the body. If the animal is then castrated before the testosterone affects the hypothalamus, an important change takes place. Although the animal has a male body, it does not behave sexually as a male. The hypothalamus, which ultimately controls the body's endocrine functions, remains female.

To prove that, researchers have removed an ovary from a healthy female rat and implanted it into a male which had been castrated at birth. They found that the ovary continued to function in normal female cycles. It could do that only because, as in the female, the pituitary of the castrated male rat secreted the hormones necessary in cyclic fashion rather than continuously, as in males. And the pituitary's behavior was a direct response to orders from the hypothalamus, which, uninfluenced by testosterone, functioned in the normal female manner.

Apparently testosterone prevents the "female" part of the hypothalamus from developing. All this suggests a few assumptions:

—The psychobiological homosexual cannot be changed through testosterone administration in childhood, adolescence, or adulthood, and probably not after the first few months of fetal life. Testosterone *does* have an affect on homosexuals. It sometimes acts as an aphrodisiac, particularly in the sex centers of the nonmasculinized hypothalamus. But it does not change their sexual orientation. (Please see Appendix, page 213.)

—Brain surgery cannot specifically reduce homosexuality. Among the many cases to support that statement are seven reported by Professor Hans Orthner of the University Department of Neurology at Göttingen. Orthner's patients were men with a compulsive urge to molest boys. Each of the men was in extreme social and legal difficulties. For example, the first man to achieve the operation had spent three terms in jail and had been declared a public menace by the courts. He had been diagnosed as a psychopathic homosexual with egocentric behavior and autistic-schizophrenic traits, and his electroencephalogram readings were abnormal.

The operation involved destroying by electric shock the portion of the hypothalamus believed to regulate the sex urge. The result is what Orthner and his colleagues call a "social recovery." The patient remains out of trouble and out of jail. He is not cured of his homosexuality per se, for he still has no interest in the opposite sex. He has simply lost his sex drive. Often the operation leads to impotence. Those who undergo it become apathetic and may suffer side effects such as disturbance of visual memory. Antiandrogenic drugs would have virtually the same effect while avoiding the potential risks of so dangerous an operation.

—Psychosexual development, like physical development, occurs not in either/or fashion, but along a sliding scale upon which there are no arbitrary marks to distinguish the normal from the abnormal. No one with the slightest insight into the homosexual community would accept as true the frequently made claim that homosexual behavior is merely a matter of preference. Just as a heterosexual man has a compulsion, often quite beyond his control, to mate with women, so the biological homosexual is *driven* to sexual relations with men. He is in the minority. He fails to propagate the species. He is, on occasion, noticeably lacking in masculine bearing and traits. Yet he fits with perfect harmony into that sliding scale of masculinity, and it is in fact inconceivable that in the normal course of things there would not develop a great many homosexuals.

Shortly after Dr. Kolodny published his study showing a decrease of testosterone among male homosexuals, he and the renowned Dr. William Masters held a press conference. There the two experts agreed that low testosterone levels might not incline toward homosexuality after all, but perhaps the reverse was true. The homosexual life-style might in some way keep testosterone levels low. Subsequent studies have shown, as we have seen, that there is probably no link between sex preferences and testosterone levels, but one well-known homosexual was willing to agree that the homosexual life might keep testosterone levels down. Astronomer Franklin E. Kameny, president of the Mattachine Society of Washington, D.C., said,

> On the basis that homosexuals are likely to be more sexually active than heterosexuals, I'm wondering if a nagging, low-level subliminal frustration in the heterosexual might not contribute to the difference in plasma testosterone levels. Remember the studies showing that when men have been away from women for a long time, on shipboard, their beard growth rates increase when they near port in anticipation. In certain conditions, the heterosexual may have his testosterone levels driven up, rather than the homosexual's being driven down.

Widely accepted is the assertion that homosexuals are far more active sexually than are their heterosexual counterparts. In fact, the ancient Greek, Soranus, recognized that and wrote,

> The fact is that, although the practices of such persons are unnatural to human beings, lust overcomes modesty and puts to shameful use parts intended for other functions. That is, in the case of certain individuals, there is no limit to their desire and no hope of satisfying it; and they cannot be content with their own lot (heterosexuality), the lot which divine providence had marked out for them in assigning definite functions to the parts of the body.*

Even in childhood, according to Dr. I. Bieber, New York psychiatrist and well-known author, ". . . homosexuals were more often excessively preoccupied with sexuality. . . ." According to research by Dr. Martin Manosevitz reported in the February,

*From Caelius Aurelianus, *On Acute Diseases and On Chronic Diseases*, ed. and trans. by I. E. Drabkin (Chicago: University of Chicago Press, 1950).

1972, issue of the *Journal of Sex Research,* the homosexuals he interviewed began masturbating at twelve and a half years of age, while heterosexuals began almost a year later. The homosexuals ejaculated earlier, had earlier and more frequent sex fantasies, and began sexual relationships with others at an earlier age.

Studies by Marcel T. Saghir, MD, of the department of psychiatry at Washington University School of Medicine in St. Louis, show that at no age were the heterosexual men as sexually active as the homosexual. The homosexuals also masturbated almost twice as often as the heterosexuals.

Perhaps the biological homosexual is, like the female, erotically hyperresponsive to testosterone, that produced by his own testes. Sexual compulsion is not only the result of this hypothalamic orientation, however; the compulsion also reinforces the homosexuality since homosexual partners are usually available more quickly and with less complexity of involvement.

If society should ever determine for some reason that there is particular value in making homosexuality extinct, it will have to recognize, the hallowed tenets of psychotherapy notwithstanding, that homosexuals are no more likely than heterosexuals to be converted from their particular desires and gratifications. The orientation must be prevented, not reversed, and that means an enormous amount of research into fetal hormone production and manipulation. Certainly sexual attitudes can be programmed in the fetus. It has already been done in laboratory animals.

But there is a far more significant question at stake here—not *can* it be done? but *should* it be? Says Franklin Kameny, "We have a moral right to become, to be, and to remain as we are. How we got that way doesn't matter in the least." While homosexuality may be a *social* abnormality, it is biologically a natural development along the scale from femininity to masculinity. The homosexual is as much a normal product of nature as is the rugged hyperheterosexual, or the man so involved in a career that he is practically asexual. Each of these conditions is a deviation from the commonplace. And, biologically speaking, that is just about all they are.

15

Testosterone and the Prostate

Whether or not testosterone causes prostate cancer is a question that virtually screams for an answer, for many doctors hesitate to prescribe the hormone for men over fifty-five, regardless of the need, precisely because they are concerned that there may be a relationship. Their hesitation is understandable for prostate cancer is a very serious matter. More than any other organ of a man's body, including his lungs, the prostate has that particular tendency to become malignant. If it is discovered in the early stages, the cure rate is high. But at that point there may be no symptoms. The disease can be discovered only by a rectal examination in which a doctor finds a hard lump or nodule on the prostate's surface. The chances the lump will be malignant are about 50 percent.

No doctor wants to risk increasing those odds by prescribing a drug that he suspects, for whatever reason, may be responsible for contributing to that grave disease.

The assumption that testosterone contributes to prostate cancer seems logical enough on the surface. As we have discussed, the male hormone is responsible for the growth of *all* male sex organs, and that includes the prostate. An adolescent who, for any reason, is incapable of testosterone production will have a small, undeveloped prostate throughout life. If he is given testosterone supplementation, the prostate will enlarge to normal size. There is no question that testosterone is essential to prostatic growth. It is easy to understand how one might make the assumption that, since testosterone is necessary for normal prostatic growth, too much of the hormone might cause wild, uncontrolled growth—cancer.

In 1941, two researchers, C. Hoggins and C. V. Hodges, presented evidence to support that conclusion in the journal, *Cancer Research* (I, 293-297). These researchers reported on three patients whose prostate cancers enlarged when they were treated with testosterone. Since that time a couple of similar reports have appeared in the medical literature.

But these were all cases in which the hormone seemed to enhance the growth of a tumor which already existed, rather than cause cancer in the first place. Today few would seriously argue that testosterone actually caused any cancer to develop, for there is no evidence whatever to indicate that. But numerous authorities point to the studies cited to prove that testosterone exacerbates already existing cancers. For that reason one of the most common conservative approaches to carcinoma of the prostate is castration. Often it is done chemically rather than surgically—a drug is given which prevents testosterone from being absorbed into the tissue cells. Such drugs are called antiandrogens. Often estrogen is also given, since, as we have said, it competes with testosterone, elevating the levels of the sex hormone binding globulin, which traps the male hormone. Used together, these approaches virtually eliminate testosterone from the body.

The theory is that the gland will shrink and shrivel. That is a natural, predictable response to starvation of the essential hormonal nutrient, since all the organs of our bodies are constantly losing old cells and replacing them with new ones. If the building materials for the new cells are not available, the organ will necessarily shrink.

That castration, either surgical or chemical, improves the health of a prostate cancer victim at least temporarily is beyond doubt. The entire organ, including the tumor, shrinks, sometimes spectacularly. If, as often happens, the cancer has spread to the bones, causing serious pain, the suffering will be reduced. The patient will be more cheerful, begin eating better, and gain weight.

But, says Dr. John T. Grayhack, "Hormone therapy is considered a palliative measure, providing long-term control of neoplasm (cancer) in some patients and very little control in others." Neither castration nor estrogen therapy ever provides a cure, and in 20 to 30 percent of all cases, it does not restrain the tumor's growth at all.

Writing in the new medical text, *Male Accessory Sex Organs*, Grayhack makes another significant point: "No convincing evidence of superiority of orchiectomy (castration) or administration of one of the variety of available estrogens as initial therapy has been presented.... Unequivocal evidence that hormonal treatment of patients with carcinoma of the prostate increased the length as well as the quality of survival has not been presented."

True, there has been shrinkage. True, pain and other symptoms have been temporarily alleviated. Yet there is no conclusive evidence that either a longer or more pleasant life resulted.

According to Patrick McGrady, former science editor of the American Cancer Society, the improvement resulting from hormone therapy is brief—less than a year on average, occasionally three or four years, and in a few more than a decade.

Some therapists assumed the cancer grew again because other endocrine glands increased testosterone production to meet the demands for the hormone. Their solutions included surgically removing the adrenals and the pituitary. The procedure did little more than throw the entire endocrine system into chaos.

So, not only is there no evidence that testosterone *causes* prostate cancer, but it may not even contribute to the tumor's growth. Yet there may be a relationship between testosterone and prostate cancer after all—an inverse relationship. There is some reason to believe that it is the *decreasing* testosterone production that accompanies aging in men which encourages abnormal prostatic growth.

Now let us do some supposing. A man has reached fifty-five

and, predictably, his testosterone production has started dropping. Prostate cells have begun to deteriorate, their nuclei becoming deformed. Many of the tiny mitochondria in each cell vanish. The mitochondria are the bodies which utilize glucose and oxygen to produce the cells' (and the body's) energy. The network of material surrounding the nucleus changes and seems to age or degenerate. The tiny vacuoles (cisternae and vesicles which serve as the cell's reservoir of water and oil) apparently wither and collapse.

In the more seriously degenerated cells, the lysosomes, or the cells' janitors, have already begun cleaning out the debris. It is a job lysosomes do throughout our lives to make room for new, healthy cells. But we must remember that healthy prostate cells cannot be produced in any great quantity by most men at this stage of life because of decreasing testosterone production. As endocrinologist Dieter Kirchheim points out, in both their development and activity prostatic cells are greatly dependent on testosterone. "For example," writes Kirchheim in *Male Accessory Sex Organs*, "synthesis of protein and vital nucleic acids and enzyme levels in the prostate are under the control of androgens (primarily testosterone), which are also fundamental for the development and maintenance of the apparatus for the synthesis of proteins, i.e., the ribosomes and rough endoplasmic reticulum. . . ." With testosterone levels continuing to fall after age fifty-five, the average prostate would simply undergo senile atrophy—the ordinary wasting away of cells because of old age.

Then something quite unexplainable happens. New cells spring into existence, large and youthful. But they are not normal prostate cells—they cannot carry on all the functions the older cells did. And they are not only youthful, but apparently immature. The mitochondria do not work properly. The enzyme secretions are not what they should be. Such problems are to be expected for these new cells have been formed from the deformed nuclei of the older ones. The chromosomal instructions have undoubtedly been damaged through degeneration.

No one knows why those aging prostate cells spring to new life, and *that is the crucial question.* Our supposition is that these aging cells, which, like all living organisms, will adapt to their environment in order to maintain survival, undergo a kind of mutation. Ultimately they, and the new cells to which they give birth, no longer require testosterone for growth. The new cells in particular are marvelously healthy, obviously not starved of a hormone essential to them.

According to our supposition, we would expect to see cancer developing first in that portion of the prostate earliest deprived of testosterone, for if the atrophying cells did not mutate into cancer cells with no testosterone requirement, they would die. And indeed, 80 percent of prostate cancers arise in the portion of the gland which is quickest to undergo senile atrophy. Dr. Kirchheim says there is evidence that "cancer cells may originate from prostatic cells that have previously undergone senile atrophy, and that cancer cells fail to attain maturity which is normally mediated through androgenic stimulation."

That statement may be of profound importance for what Kirchheim seems to suggest is that, if sufficient testosterone were present at the crucial time, those immature cancer cells might well develop into mature, healthy, and normal prostate cells rather than deadly cancers.

If testosterone deficiency causes prostate cells to mutate into cancer cells, we would also expect any testosterone still being secreted to find use in the remaining normal aging prostate cells. When a major testosterone source is eliminated, through chemical or surgical castration or estrogen therapy, normal prostate cells would certainly atrophy, causing a measurable shrinkage in the gland as a whole, including the tumor. But unlike the normal cells, the malignant ones have the capacity to adapt to testosterone deprivation. It may take them months, or even years, to begin flourishing in a total absence of testosterone, but eventually they will do so.

Once again the theory that prostate cells mutate to survive without testosterone is supported by the evidence: Chemical castration and estrogen administration do not cure prostate cancer. They merely delay its growth (presumably until the mutant cells begin flourishing).

The hypothesis becomes ever more intriguing for it suggests that testosterone, if given early enough in life (perhaps the middle forties to fifties), may actually prevent prostatic senile atrophy, and thus malignancy. That possibility has not apparently been investigated, but some researchers have gone a step further and attempted to repeat the experiments of Hoggins and Hodges. In contrast to the original discouraging results showing that prostate cancer grows more rapidly following testosterone supplementation, modern investigators have found conflicting results.

Two of the researchers are George R. Prout, Jr., MD, and Walter R. Brewer, MD, of the Medical College of Virginia and the University of Miami School of Medicine respectively. They administered testosterone to twenty-six men with the two most serious stages of prostate cancer. The therapy lasted only three to thirty-three days, and in no case was any measurable improvement noticed. But when these patients were compared with a control group receiving estrogen therapy, the researchers state, the responses were roughly equivalent. The one exception was a man receiving testosterone.

C.J.S. was seventy-six years old and terminally ill with prostate cancer. He entered the hospital with severe back pain, weakness, and complete loss of appetite. As a result, his weight had fallen to eighty-nine pounds. His prostate had been enlarging rapidly and he could not sit without assistance because of the pain.

By that time he had suffered prostate cancer for five years. He had undergone transurethral resection to remove urethral pressure, and he had also been castrated and was given estrogens.

The fact that he had survived for five years indicates the tumor growth had been temporarily arrested. Then suddenly it flared up again, with cancer cells spreading to the skull, spine, and other bones. Through rectal examination large nodules could be felt on the prostate itself.

The man was given testosterone three times weekly for a month. In that short time his pain vanished, he was able to move around without help, and his weight increased to 112 pounds. The improvement was so marked that he was dismissed from the hospital and treated as an outpatient for six months. By then the tumor had once again impinged upon the urethra and another transurethral resection was required. Thereafter, the patient gained thirty more pounds, a significant sign that he was feeling better and that his health was improved. He was virtually without symptoms of the cancer. The nodules that had developed in the prostate were no longer palpable.

But the cancer cells were still detectable by x-ray in the bones, and almost a year after the testosterone therapy began, the man was back in the hospital with severe back and hip pain. Then the prostate tumor began enlarging again and, not long after, the man died.

Considering that the doctors expected his death almost a year earlier than it occurred, his improvement was remarkable indeed. Yet too much ought not to be made of this particular case since the patient proved remarkable in the first place by surviving the initial five years after the cancer was diagnosed. What's more, the testosterone may have provided a sense of well-being through its known functions—encouraging bone growth, protein utilization, increased muscle mass (weight), and even a more optimistic outlook.

Yet other researchers have reported definite improvement with testosterone therapy, and still others have shown that testosterone at least did not enhance tumor growth.

Herbert Kupperman, a doctor who regularly prescribes testosterone to older men, was asked in a recent *Medical World News* interview, "What is the association between hormone therapy and prostate cancer?" Kupperman replied:

> Of the hundred fifty males I've treated, I haven't had one case of prostatic cancer.... if I was doing anything that was accelerating the rate of growth of the cancer, I would expect that this would be appearing....
>
> Another point is that cancer of the prostate seems to be a disease that affects the older individual, by and large the individual past the climacteric. If cancer of the prostate was due to an androgenic stimulus, why then would it wait until androgen levels are at their lowest ebb, rather than at their peak, in the normal male? When you have a cancer that supposedly responds to gonadal hormones, you really wonder sometimes whether the hormones are etiological (the

cause of a disease) or beneficial. The incidence of cancer in males, as in cancer of the breast in females, might be lower (in those treated with hormones) than that expected in the population as a whole.

At least four processes take place in the average man after age fifty-five:

—Blood and urine testosterone levels fall, and studies show that it is because there are fewer active interstitial cells.

—Sex hormone binding globulin levels rise, binding testosterone, and thus compounding the deficiency in free testosterone available to the body.

—Estrogen levels, which remain stable until the fifth decade of life, increase steadily and rapidly thereafter.

—Changes begin taking place in the prostate. Fibrous tissue develops, enzyme production decreases, and cells begin to atrophy.

Is the key to prostate cancer buried in those facts? Or might it be, as some researchers suggest, that certain environmental pollutants known to cause cancer, and which are chemically similar to testosterone, are utilized by aging and defective prostate cells to support renewed, uncontrolled growth? Such questions are not impossible to answer, but because they still go begging, seventeen thousand men a year die of prostate cancer. They are for the most part old men—nine out of every ten in the United States are seventy years of age or more. And since old men die anyway, there is perhaps a bit less concern and a bit less willingness to fund essential research necessary to put prostate cancer into the same grave as polio and smallpox and other once dread diseases.

Until that is done, the sensible man will take no chances. From his forties on he will seek regular prostate examinations. Twice a year is not too often. Fortunately, rectal examinations are very effective in identifying the nodules of early prostate cancer. Diagnosed and treated in the early stages, most victims can survive. When the cancer is not discovered until the final stage—and that happens *most* of the time—only five or six percent survive.

Regarding testosterone therapy, there is no medical reason

that any man, whatever his age, should be denied it. In summary, the male hormone does not cause cancer, and, in fact, its *decline* after middle age may be a factor in the development of prostatic malignancy. Although eliminating all testosterone may produce a temporary regression in cancer that already exists, the cancer will not be cured. In cases where the cancer already exists, the findings are completely contradictory. Some studies say testosterone supplementation will stimulate the cancer. Others say precisely the opposite—that the malignancy will decrease. At this point there has not been sufficient research to establish a convincing argument either way.

16

Too Much of a Good Thing

Some years ago newspapers throughout the country told the story of a nine-year-old Brooklyn boy who had suffered enlarged tonsils, allergies, and continuous colds. The family's enterprising physician determined for some unexplainable reason to treat those symptoms with testosterone. The parents filed a million-dollar lawsuit against him, claiming "the boy has acquired all the characteristics and sex attributes of a mature male and has since then been afflicted by a strong sex urge."

The point of that story and this chapter is that testosterone is in no sense a panacea. It is a potent and essential hormone, and even a slight deficiency in it can sometimes have far-reaching effects on the body's capacity to function normally. But obviously there are many physical functions uninfluenced by testosterone. What's more, an excess can, in at least some cases, prove a decided disadvantage.

One example is the case of the nine-year-old boy. Any young boy given sufficient testosterone will promptly mature physically and develop a libido, or sex urge. He will undergo all the changes he would normally experience at adolescence—his sex organs will enlarge, he will develop body hair, muscle mass, and usually a deepening voice. Most important, and probably most deleterious in the long run, the bones of his body will cease lengthening. Thus, depending on the amount of hormone he receives and the age at which it is administered, he may go through life significantly shorter than other men.

Women, too, are sometimes adversely affected by testosterone. It is prescribed for women with breast cancer for the same reason that estrogen is given for controlling prostate tumors. Almost always some virilization takes place. (The women are then said to be hirsute.) Rarely a tumor of the adrenal gland might produce hirsutism in both men and women. Thus the bearded lady of the sideshow is no laughing matter, for if the beard and body hair are real, there is a good chance the woman has a tumor.

What appears to be normal testosterone levels in some men may be excessive in others, at least from a social viewpoint. Criminologists have for many years asserted a link between male hormones and certain types of criminal behavior. We have already discussed castration as therapy for sex deviates. Surgery is not as common today as is the use of drugs such as cyproterone acetate, an androgen antagonist. During the past two decades a great many sex offenders have requested these antiandrogen drugs. In virtually all cases the therapy has reduced the libido, which is not to say that it converted pederasts, sadists, rapists, exhibitionists, and such to the so-called norm of society. It simply reduced their sex drives to the point where they were *inactive* pederasts, sadists, and so forth.

(A curious paradox: Cyproterone acetate does not cause a decrease in testosterone production. In fact, the drug seems to encourage higher blood testosterone levels. Apparently the antiandrogen drugs work by "impersonating" male hormones, persuading the receptor proteins which usher the hormone into the target cells to link up with the antiandrogens instead. Since the receptors are kept busy with the impostor, they have no time for the true hormone, and it remains in the blood unused.)

Recent studies suggest that not only sex offenders, but other criminals with a greater than normal tendency to violence and aggressiveness, may have an excess of testosterone, at least for them. Twenty-one prisoners nineteen to thirty-two years old had their testosterone levels analyzed frequently for two weeks. Then those figures were compared with their criminal behavior from childhood through age eighteen. Only ten of the twenty-one had committed aggressive, physically violent crimes such as murder, attempted murder, assault, and armed robbery. Precisely those ten men had significantly higher testosterone levels than did the eleven others who had committed routine offenses such as car theft and burglary.

That study found no relationship between testosterone levels and psychological test reports of hostility, aggressiveness, or anxiety. But another study, one by Dr. Harold Persky and his colleagues at the Division of Endocrinology and Reproduction, Albert Einstein Medical Center, Philadelphia, found highly significant correlations between those characteristics and testosterone levels, particularly in younger men.

Certainly there is no evidence to suggest that testosterone *compels* a man to be violent or hostile. To make a very rough analogy, testosterone is a tool, a hammer. One man will use it to build a house, another to tear one down, and a third as a weapon of assault. The hammer itself is in no case responsible. Still, by removing the tool, the danger is reduced.

As some researchers put it, testosterone acts *permissively*. It allows the man already inclined toward violence and hostility to act out those tendencies. Perhaps it actually prods him to do so. But there is no evidence to suggest that the man who is socially well-integrated will become otherwise under testosterone's influence.

The objection to antiandrogen therapy for the criminally violent or hostile is that it has the same effects as castration. Even more quickly than through surgery, the accessory sex glands begin to shrink and degenerate. The hypothalamus, no longer stimulated by the hormone, ceases to signal sexual compulsion, and, presumably, aggressiveness. Unlike surgical castration, however, the drugs' effects can be eliminated within a few weeks simply by discontinuing their use.

Too much testosterone can also be hazardous to health in some cases. Drug companies are required by law to warn prescribing physicians that prolonged testosterone administration can cause salt and water retention in the body's tissues. That can add stress to the heart and kidneys—stress that damaged organs may not be capable of withstanding.

Very rare are these additional testosterone side effects which the pharmaceutical companies are required to make known: hypersensitivity reactions, including rash and dermatitis; local irritation, redness, and pain when injections are used; decrease in sperm and ejaculatory volume; gynecomastia; a violent allergic reaction to the testosterone as a foreign substance not produced in the body; and priapism (prolonged, painful erection not related to sex desire).

But testosterone may have a far more fundamental negative influence on male health than is generally recognized. It might be the spring in the time clock that has limited him since the beginning of written history to the biblical three-score-and-ten-year life span.

Males have traditionally lived fewer years than females have. Some explanations for that are obvious. Men fought and died in wars. Men took greater risks. Even driving to and from work during his employed lifetime exposed a man to about 21,600 opportunities for an automobile accident.

Comparatively shorter life expectancy for the male is not a phenomenon unique to humans. In fact, among both vertebrates and invertebrates, with few exceptions, the female outlives the male. In eight different strains of mice the male life span was shorter than the female's by 0.1 to 2.4 months, in life cycles which lasted from 11.1 to 21.7 months. Female rats live about 773 days, while the males live only 712 days. In another strain the females lived 687 days; the males 622. Those studies and others show a consistent difference in life spans of about 10 percent, roughly the same as that in humans.

As long ago as 1948 endocrinology researcher Dr. J. B. Hamilton theorized, in *Recent Progress in Hormone Research*, that the difference in longevity resulted from the higher testosterone levels in males. Some years later he tested his hypothesis by comparing a series of castrated male cats with normal ones. The castrates lived 8.8 years; the normal 7.7. But that study was set up in a way that gave an advantage to the castrates.

Recently a much more careful and complicated study was conducted at Cornell University. The subjects consisted of eleven groups of fifty rats each—castrated males and females, normal rodents, virgins, sexually experienced, and others castrated with implanted testosterone and estrogen. When all the mice had died, the tallied scores showed virtually no statistically significant differences in life span. The one exception, according to researcher S. A. Asdell of Cornell University's Animal Science Department: "Rats exposed to their own or implanted estrogens had a longer average life span than did those exposed to their own or to implanted testosterone."

The evidence that testosterone is in some way related to the shorter male life span is quite convincing, but it raises a larger question than it answers: Just how does testosterone have that effect? A couple of generations ago people were quite content to believe that an individual in his sixties or seventies simply died of old age. The concept was that death is an intrinsic part of life, a notion still expressed on occasion in religious and philosophical circles. The fact is that the body wages awesome and indescribably violent war against death, sometimes crippling itself, sometimes accidentally destroying itself in the process. People do not die because that is simply the way life goes. They die because certain normal and essential functions cease.

Testosterone, if it causes the shortened life span of a male, does so through the channels which cause his death, primarily cardiovascular disease (heart attacks and strokes). Apparently testosterone, through its influence on the male personality, compels him to undertake certain types of stress, and this contributes to a shortened male life span. Some men work under continual deadline pressures. Others are in constant conflict with other personalities, scolding, badgering, or being scolded and badgered. Still others are called upon to make decisions on a regular basis, and a mistake may not only prove expensive to their companies, but may put their jobs in jeopardy. Historically, women usually did not face this type of stress. Some men shrugged it off. Others developed ulcers, high blood pressure, and heart disease.

A good deal has been written during the last few years about the personality traits of the men who are most susceptible to stress-related heart disease.

Apparently 90 percent of men who have heart attacks have the same personality traits. They are impatient, busy, accumulating things instead of being content with themselves; they always feel compelled to be rushing and doing things; they have nervous gestures such as teeth grinding and fist clenching; and they suffer guilt when they are not accomplishing something. Sometimes they are referred to as Type A personalities; they do not notice changes in landscapes, buildings, or rooms. Friends could grow mustaches or shave them off, and Type A would not notice. Their wives could move furniture or even redecorate, and it would hardly make an impression.

Although the cardiac-prone personality is common among executives, factory workers may have the same characteristics. In fact, about 50 percent of all American males are probably Type A.

According to cardiologists Mayer Friedman and Ray H. Rosenman, authors of *Type A Behavior and Your Heart* (Knopf, 1974),

> In the absence of Type A behavior patterning, coronary heart disease almost never occurs before seventy years of age, regardless of the fatty foods eaten, the cigarettes smoked, or the lack of exercise. But when this behavior pattern is present, coronary heart disease can easily erupt in one's thirties or forties. We are convinced that the spread of Type A behavior explains why death by heart disease, once confined mainly to the elderly, is becoming increasingly common among younger people.

The fact is that most men are not killed while commuting to work, and relatively few die in war. It is the male testosterone-stimulated personality which is responsible for the fact that a woman born between 1939 and 1941 can expect to live 67.3 years, while the average life expectancy for a man born in that period is only 62.8 years.

A couple of solutions exist. The first, castration, is not likely to gain many followers, particularly among the aggressive, hard-driving men whose life spans would be most benefited. The second alternative is a very definite effort to change personality characteristics. That is the most difficult step, but it has been done by many men, particularly when their health has been threatened by cardiovascular disease symptoms.

Perhaps the final solution rests with endocrinology research. It is possible that one of these days investigators will learn the mechanism whereby testosterone creates the Type A personality and will find ways to moderate the effects produced on the body by the resulting stress. The chances are good that when we learn how to prevent heart attacks, the answer will come not from the cardiologists but from the endocrinologists.

17

The Active Life of a Testis

The testosterone administered or prescribed by a physician is a drug manufactured from cholesterol in a factory. As with all drugs, it has its disadvantages, and we discussed some of them in the previous chapter. There are other, more prosaic ones: Drugs cost money, as do doctors' visits. There is also some inconvenience in relying regularly upon a drug.

With testosterone there is another disadvantage: Chronic testosterone supplementation will cause the testes to decrease hormone production, perhaps finally ceasing their function entirely. The reason for that is easy to understand. If the hypothalamus receives the message that blood testosterone levels are high, it signals the pituitary to stop sending gonadotrophins to the testes. Without these pituitary hormones the testes will not function.

Most people know that a muscle which is not used atrophies. (For example, when an arm or leg is kept in a cast for a few months.) It literally wastes away. The same occurs in unused testicles. That is no cause for concern in older men whose testes have already atrophied. The hormone can only be a blessing, for the damage is already done. The same is true of younger men whose testes are damaged, and the chances of regeneration are nil. What's more, when the testes are healthy to start with, discontinuation of testosterone therapy often leads to a rebound response, the same as occurs with sperm production—eventually the testes may begin producing testosterone again at pretherapy levels. That is common, but it is not certain.

For men who, for one reason or another, seek an alternative to synthetic testosterone, the following chapters offer some important information. There are several steps almost any man can take to increase his own testosterone production as well as to eliminate, or at least recognize, testosterone antagonists in his environment.

Some men, undoubtedly without realizing it, have taken precisely these steps. While averages overall show a significant decrease in testosterone levels after the age of fifty-five, in some men there is no such reduction, or it is so slight as to be completely insignificant. Such cases are not common, nor are they extremely rare. For some thus far unexplained reason their testes go right on producing youthful amounts of sperm and hormones into their sixties, seventies, and eighties.

It is surprising and disappointing that these men have not been studied thoroughly, for in their continuing capacity to maintain hormone production into old age may reside the key to unlocking the same capability for all men.

Certainly the body's functions are to a great extent genetically determined. Our size and shape, our bone structure, musculature, and even our capacity to think are to a degree the products of our genes. But that influence is obviously not even remotely the exclusive definition of our potential. Olympic athletes are born into families whose genealogy offers not the slightest suggestion of superior athletic capability. In general the same can be said of intellectual genius and artistic talent. While heredity provides the capacity, environment permits the achievement.

Some men may be genetically predisposed to producing glandular secretions well into old age, but there is increasing and convincing evidence that it is the life-style, rather than extraordinary natural endowment, which allows one man in every couple of dozen to maintain youthful testosterone levels throughout his life. One of these factors seems to be physical exercise. That is a conclusion of a study undertaken by J. R. Sutton and his colleagues at the Garvan Institute of Medical Research, St. Vincent's Hospital, Sydney, Australia, and published in the *British Medical Journal* on March 3, 1973. The team studied two groups of athletes—fourteen oarsmen of a rowing team and seven swimmers. These were not typical college athletes, but highly trained men who had achieved Olympic standards. The training was rigid, involving two sessions daily—one all-out and another somewhat less demanding.

Sutton tested blood testosterone levels for all the men before and after each of the two sessions. He found that when the exercise was less than maximal, there was no change in testosterone levels, but when the physical effort was all-out, blood testosterone increased dramatically.

Dr. Sutton questioned whether the result had something to do with the exceptional physical fitness of the subjects, rather than the exercise itself, in which case it would have no application to the testosterone production of ordinary men. To determine that, he selected four more subjects—medical students in good health, but not athletes. He had them exercise for twenty minutes on a stationary bicycle, and he collected blood samples before, during, and after the performance. After ten minutes of activity, testosterone levels began to rise, reaching their peak at twenty minutes, when the exercise was discontinued. (They would possibly have gone higher had the activity continued.)

Of course there is good reason to expect hormone levels to rise during exercise. For one thing, studies show that exercising muscles have an increased capacity to store energy in the form of glycogen, but to do so they need increased amounts of testosterone. The hormone may also increase carbohydrate metabolism in muscles, thereby helping to meet the increased demand for energy. In both cases the greater need for testosterone would stimulate increased production.

The testosterone/exercise link was predictable, for other researchers had already shown that exercise triggers increased blood levels of growth hormone, cortisol, and other hormones. There was no reason to expect the testes to behave differently from other endocrine glands. Two findings were curious, however:

—There was no increase in the amount of hormone bound by the sex hormone binding globulin, so that the increased testosterone was free to virilize the men.

—There was no rise in the pituitary gonadotrophins which stimulate the testes to produce testosterone. Thus the extreme exercise was in some way permitting the testes to operate more efficiently on their own.

To repeat a point made earlier, testosterone secretions are highly dependent upon blood flow surrounding the testes. Studies made more than a decade ago have established that. The hormone is secreted through the walls of the glands directly into the blood. If it is not swept away through an adequate blood flow, apparently this "crowding" of testosterone molecules backs up within the glands, relaying to the interstitial cells the message to reduce production. Whether that theory is precisely correct or not, the fact is that the decreased blood flow produces decreased testosterone production. Exercise increases blood flow.

Exercise also causes the adrenal glands to secrete more hormones, and some of them, particularly noradrenaline, have been shown to stimulate the synthesis and secretion of testosterone by the testes.

Another phenomenon related to exercise: Less blood flows through the liver during strenuous physical activity. The logical assumption is that less testosterone is therefore metabolized to weaker forms.

This jungle of technical explanation has its importance, but it also tends to smother the obvious, the fact that continuing more or less strenuous physical activity has a health-maintaining effect upon the body. Says Dr. Lawrence Rarick of the University of Wisconsin, "Studies of German men who were athletic in their youth indicate that continuation of a physically active life can postpone many of the symptoms of aging by as much as twenty to thirty years, with apparently no harmful effect on the individual." Some of these men maintained their prime throughout their sixties and seventies. "While the evidence is not clear concerning the effects of exercise on longevity," says Dr. Rarick, "there is strong support for the belief that the person will have a healthier, happier, and more productive span of years late in life by including a regular program of physical activity in his regimen of living."

Innumerable authorities agree. Says Dr. Henry J. Montoye of Michigan State University, "There is no question in my mind that regular exercise of the proper intensity and duration can do much to postpone the deterioration which commonly occurs as the individual becomes older. There are all kinds of cases in the sports world where amazing physical feats have been performed by people well up in years."

Says Dr. Lawrence E. Morehouse of the University of California, "A person who has been accustomed to vigorous physical activity all of his life may still be as capable of exercise at seventy as the sedentary man of forty."

There is a widely pervasive attitude among many laymen and a few medical practitioners that as one grows older, he should by all means become less active. Fallacious as that view is, it is nonetheless understandable, considering today's machine-age thinking. Certainly as our automobile grows older, we pamper it, especially if we cannot afford a new one. We take it on fewer trips, accelerate more gently, drive slower. We realize that, little by little, that car is going to wear away. Every stroke of the piston wears another few atoms from the cylinder. Every jar of the springs stresses them further. There is no way to repair this inexorable deterioration.

We carry that analogy over to the human body, but it is patently false. Muscles, including the heart, do not deteriorate with use. Precisely the opposite is true: Stressed muscles grow stronger in order to endure additional stress. As the body grows older, it does indeed deteriorate in certain respects. But the amazing fact is that the body, unlike the automobile, is a living organism, and as such has the phenomenal capacity to adapt to new stresses, even as it ages. In fact, physical activity actually retards many symptoms of aging, in addition to reduced testosterone production.

Through experiments with several thousand men, Dr. Thomas K. Cureton, professor emeritus of the University of Illinois, has suggested that the classic symptoms of old age are merely the result of inactivity. For example:

—In the aged, fat commonly replaces muscle; exercise converts the fat to needed energy and rebuilds muscle.

—Metabolic rate decreases; exercise increases metabolism dramatically at all ages. And metabolism remains high, not for a mere few minutes, but for twelve to forty-eight hours (by which time additional exercise should be undertaken).

—Aging brings with it a loss in motor fitness—balance, flexibility, agility, and reaction time. But these are skills we are not born with. Each is learned. The baby has no sense of balance whatever, no agility, and very poor coordination and reaction time. When his muscles develop, they will not necessarily be flexible. It is only as we run and jump and climb that we learn balance. We perfect it in bicycling. Then, when we get old enough to drive a car, we discard the cycle and our sense of balance starts downhill. Yet those who have continued to use bicycles, even into their seventies, have as fine a sense of balance as they ever had. The story is the same regarding agility and reaction time. As for flexibility, it leaves people, young or old, when they fail to stretch their muscles regularly. Often aches and pains self-diagnosed as rheumatism and arthritis are merely severely stiff muscles, preventable through exercises which give them the opportunity to flex and stretch.

—Aging men can do less physical work than they could when they were younger, and this is associated with decreased oxygen uptake in the blood and ultimately the body's cells. But research by Roy J. Shephard, MD, PhD, of the University of Toronto shows that, to a great extent, this condition results from inactivity, not age. In his book, *Endurance Fitness* (University of Toronto Press, 1969), Shephard shows that by subjecting older men to endurance training exercises, such as vigorous walking, rowing, cycling, and jogging, he was able to increase dramatically the amount of oxygen they were able to utilize, thereby increasing their work capacity to that of men several years younger.

—As the average sedentary American grows older, his blood vessels lose their flexibility. Their walls tear and thicken with plaques so that the vessels themselves are narrowed and the blood must push with greater force to continue circulation. This is called peripheral resistance. The heart is forced to work harder. Blood pressure increases. Sometimes the smaller vessels are entirely blocked, and circulation to these peripheral areas of the body is cut off. Thus the poor circulation and "cold feet" of old age occur.

Far tinier than the blood vessels to the feet are the capillaries serving the testes. The gonads of most older men are critically deprived of essential oxygen and nutrients. Inevitably they atrophy.

Yet this problem of blood circulation is one of the most dramatic areas in which lifelong hard physical activity can keep the body relatively youthful. Dr. Thomas Cureton has demonstrated that vigorous exercise reduces peripheral resistance of individuals despite their age (*The Physiological Effects of Exercise Programs on Adults*, Charles C. Thomas Press, 1971). In fact, Cureton's studies have shown that there is no difference between younger men and older ones with respect to peripheral resistance when both engaged in a vigorous exercise program.

Whether or not exercise reduces cholesterol levels—which is believed to cause the plaques that build up in blood vessels—is a subject of great dispute. Some claim that there is a reduction; others claim there is not. Practically all agree, however, with Dr. Larry Golding at Kent University that cholesterol levels will not *increase* if a person is engaged in a vigorous exercise program. It seems that exercise has a stabilizing effect on cholesterol levels in most people. Many researchers, especially Dr. J. S. Skinner, now at Montreal University, have established that triglycerides (another suspect in the plaque buildup) and blood sugar levels are reduced through exercise programs that are continuous and rhythmical. Researchers have recently reported at the American College of Sports Medicine meeting held in Toronto that an exercise program must be approximately forty-five minutes long to reduce cholesterol, triglycerides, and blood sugar levels. There is also a good deal of evidence that continuous and rhythmical exercise can help reduce blood pressure. Studies conducted by Dr. Fred Kasch at San Diego State and by Doctors Rudd and Day in Boston have indicated that regular exercise programs will reduce both systolic and diastolic pressures for many people.

Regarding the exciting effect exercise can have on cardiovascular problems, Dr. Cureton says, "The most fascinating type of improvement, reflected in over a hundred graduate theses and faculty researches at the Physical Fitness Research Center at the University of Illinois, is the improvement in cardiovascular condition, with reasonable expectancy that prevention of coronary thrombosis can result, or at least be postponed." What's more, jogging, cycling, and other endurance exercises that strengthen the heart also increase the efficiency of the respiratory system and deliver more fresh blood to the cells of the testes and the rest of the body. That is especially important at a time when the cells are losing efficiency and need an even greater supply of nutrients and oxygen to keep functioning at par.

The aging suffer a progressive bone loss, or osteoporosis, which leads to a weakening and brittle skeletal system. For that reason broken bones are pathetically common among the aged. Yet they are emphatically not an inevitable aspect of growing older. Weakened bones can be traced in virtually every case to two factors—lack of exercise and poor diet.

Without exercise the body has no need for stronger bones. The function of the skeletal structure is to support the muscles and organs of the body, the clothing we cover it with, the additional weight we might add to it by lifting and shoving objects, and the stresses we might encounter in day-to-day activities. The more active we are, either through physical exercise or manual labor, the greater the strength and density of our bones. It is the pull and tug of muscles against bone that causes the production of osteoblasts, or bone-building cells. Without that stimulation no new bone cells are created.

Yet old bone is continually being broken down by other cells called osteoclasts. Thus the bones of the sedentary begin a process in their late twenties to early thirties that does not culminate for perhaps twenty or thirty years. Then the perilous weakness of the body's skeleton becomes painfully clear: aches and pains, crippling, and physical deterioration, usually diagnosed as arthritis and rheumatism.

Wide agreement exists among researchers that bone strength and density can be maintained well into old age with adequate exercise—if, of course, the nutrients required for bone-building are available. These include calcium, phosphorous, trace minerals, protein, and vitamins D, A, and C. Testosterone is also essential in bone cell production.

But one of the awesome beauties of the body is that it is a complete ecosystem in its own right. The body's need for testosterone in bone construction is a fine example. When, because of exercise, the call comes to build new bone, the testes (also because of exercise) are busy producing the needed testosterone.

18
Sex and the Sex Hormone

At first glance it seems a rather bizarre form of lovemaking. C. A. Fox and his colleagues described it recently in the *Journal of Endocrinology*. A thirty-eight-year-old man married for eleven years incorporated for several months a bloodletting ritual into his sex life. At his request, before, during, and after sexual intercourse, his wife jabbed his forearm with a needle and extracted blood.

The man (we will call him Charles Hunter since Dr. Fox failed to identify him) subjected himself to the status of a pincushion not for Eros' sake but for that of science. Each blood sample was labeled and set aside, and when the sex activities were culminated, the blood was analyzed.

Charles Hunter and his colleagues had a theory that testosterone levels were strongly influenced by the amount of sex activity in which a man engaged. In fact, a good deal of research with animals already supported that proposition. Studies with bulls and rats showed a significant elevation of the hormone in the blood following sex activity. And when a male rabbit is put into the presence of a female in heat, his testosterone concentration increases tenfold.

The same is true of monkeys. Dr. Robert Rose put four of them in separate areas with plenty of food, water, and open space. After learning what their normal or baseline testosterone levels were, he released into each area a group of female monkeys. Within minutes each of the males made it clear who was boss, and for two weeks he enjoyed a private Valhalla, eating, drinking, and making love day after day. Only those endless needles intruded upon the bliss.

Rose collected blood samples from each of the males twice a week between nine and ten A.M., and also once within twenty-four hours after they were introduced to the females. As Rose admits, the frequency was not sufficient to rule out weekly or monthly testosterone cycles. But by collecting the blood samples at the same time daily, at least the twenty-four hour cycle's influence on variations was minimized.

The difference a girl monkey makes in a boy monkey's testosterone levels is nothing short of phenomenal! The increases from baseline levels were from 109 to 247 percent, which means that, regarding testosterone levels at least, the right girl monkey can make a boy monkey twice the man he used to be. As an added check Dr. Rose put the monkeys back in separate cages. Within a week their testosterone levels fell back to baseline.

Presumably what is true of bulls, mice, rabbits, monkeys, and other animals is also true of man, but that is not always so. Charles Hunter wanted proof. So he carried out two studies in the privacy of his own bedroom. In the first, he took blood samples from himself at ten o'clock each night to establish his baseline testosterone levels. He did that for forty-five days, and during that period, whenever his wife and he had sex, he also took a blood sample before orgasm and within five minutes after. Hunter's wife, whose devotion to science undoubtedly equals his own, took both blood samples from a vein in his forearm at the crucial moments. She also processed the blood samples within thirty minutes of their collection.

The second study was similar to the first, except that two control samples were taken, one at eight A.M. and the other at eight P.M.

One of the more prosaic findings of the study was to confirm that testosterone levels are much higher in the morning than at night. On only three out of forty-three days did the level of testosterone in the evening control sample exceed that of the morning.

More important, Hunter and his wife found that sex activity and testosterone levels were as closely related in humans as in other animals. Whether they made love in the morning or at night, the hormone level increased dramatically. Since the difference between morning and evening baseline levels was great—sometimes a variation of 200 to 300 percent—sex in the evening rarely raised testosterone levels to the morning baseline. But it always raised it above the evening baseline. In both cases the amount of androgen sometimes increased by more than fifty percent.

The sample taken after sex play started but before orgasm was significantly higher than the baseline. After orgasm the hormone level climbed even higher.

Like most original studies, Fox's raises more questions than it answers. An obvious one is the immortal chicken-and-egg problem: Which came first? Does the increase in testosterone in the blood stimulate the brain, trigger the libido, and drive Hunter and his wife to the bedroom? Or does the active use of the genitals in coitus produce a physiological response in the gonads, so that higher levels of testosterone are secreted? On the one hand, Fox offers support for the latter, stating that men whose blood was analyzed while they were masturbating did not show testosterone increases comparable to Hunter's while he was making love. Says Fox, "Our present results suggest that the increase in circulating testosterone levels are likely to be associated with the act of coitus itself rather than with the desire for, or anticipation of, sexual activity."

A year after Fox wrote those words another researcher, Karl Pirke, MD, with the Max Planck Institut für Psychiatrie, Munich, took Fox to task for that conclusion. He used a study of his own to do it. He divided sixteen healthy men into two groups and showed them movies. Group A was treated to hard-core pornography, while Group B watched children's cartoons. Every fifteen minutes for three and a half hours blood samples were taken from each of the men.

Dr. Pirke added one more dimension to his study. He used penile plethysmography to determine the number and strength of erections. As anticipated, there was no testosterone increase in any of the cartoon viewers. But among those watching the sex films, all but two had significant increases, the average being 35 percent above baseline.

Pirke's study makes it clear that sexual excitement, not the sex act, triggers the rise in testosterone levels. But it is not *always* true for *all* men that sexual stimulation triggers testosterone production. Fox found that masturbating men did not have significant increases, and Pirke reported that two of his eight sex film viewers, though stimulated to erection, had no increase in testosterone. There is at least one plausible explanation.

In animals sex interest alone is almost invariably associated in males with significantly increased testosterone. Tenfold increases in testosterone in rabbits occur at the mere *presence* of female rabbits in heat. The human male, however, sometimes does not show this normal biological response, and testosterone levels are not the only area in which his reaction is not that which might be expected biologically. Psychic sexual impotence—psychological frustration of capacity to achieve erection when sexually stimulated—is a condition unique to the human male. Both the static testosterone levels and the psychic impotence may be related to a particular characteristic peculiar to human sexuality—the ability to respond intellectually to sexual activity. The man suffering psychic impotence overrides his natural biological response to an erotic situation with any number of intellectual doubts and fears. There is no longer any question that the intellect has much stronger influence on human behavior than does the sex drive, which explains the immensity of guilt surrounding most human sexual activity. Many men today can relax into the urgings of their libidos only after satisfying their intellects concerning a host of questions about morality, ethics, logistics, short- and long-term implications and the more immediate strategy of approach—and whether the prospective partner stimulates any erotic interest after all.

Considering the extent to which the intellect overrides the sex drive in modern man, it is not surprising that potency problems develop, but rather that normal coitus ever takes place. It does so, in fact, because there is another side to the intellect/libido coin: Unlike most intelligent animals, man can utilize his intellect to stimulate a previously nonexistent sex drive. He does that for any number of reasons. Perhaps his partner desires sex activity. Or the man himself may be bored or lonely. Some men follow sex activity schedules, once a day every day (or whatever), whether they feel like it or not.

Such an approach to sex is less than biological in the basic sense, and it requires a synthetic stimulation. In man the intellect has come to its own rescue through the act of fantasy. Through reading erotic literature and watching films of others engaging in sex activity he literally creates in himself a desire for sexual gratification similar to that experienced by those with whom he is identifying. Sex films and literature are not used to satisfy a sex urge. Orgasm alone does that. Pornography is used as a tool of the intellect to whet the sex appetite at a time when biologically sexual tension has not built to the point at which release is essential.

"Straight away," says Desmond Morris, "we can see that there is much more intense sexual activity in our own species than in any other primate, including our closest relations." Clearly, the naked ape is the sexiest primate alive, and it is because of his unique capacity to *pursue* sexual stimulation intellectually. Thus, through sex films, fantasies, books, or direct manual stimulation of the genitals, man alone of all species routinely thrusts upon himself a desire for sex and then gratifies that desire. Biologically he is not so sexual as his sex activity indicates. But as we have already suggested, sex means a great deal more to the male Homo sapiens than it does to other animals. It offers an excuse for physical closeness, an alternative to boredom, and an assurance of manhood, of youth, of attractiveness. It offers relaxation from tension and a momentary distraction from problems. Some men claim it is even the ideal motivation to exercise.

As long as society continues to create the onslaught of emotional needs which are so well assuaged by sex activity, the various forms of libido-stimulating pornography are doing an invaluable service to society. Sometimes, however, the *soma* (body) does not keep up with the *psyche*. Fox's masturbating men, apparently responding to instructions and a synthetic stimulant to eroticism, produced no increase in testosterone levels. Two of Pirke's eight subjects viewing the sex film also failed to demonstrate an increase in testosterone.

The point is that in man, as opposed to other animals, the intellect plays an overriding role in sexual activity. Men with practically no testicular function whatever have been found on occasion to have very active sex lives, while others with high testosterone levels have been comparatively inactive. The difference is explained by individual capacity to utilize the tangible pornography as well as the intangible sex fantasy to achieve self-stimulation.

Can sex activity lead to continuing high testosterone levels? The answer is almost certainly yes. Studies show that hormone levels reach their peak an hour to an hour and a half after initial erotic stimulation and remain high for twelve to forty-eight hours. There is no evidence that the testosterone upsurge fails as man grows older.

According to several researchers, including the famed Dr. William Masters and Virginia Johnson, a highly active and continuing sex life in the younger years is related to continuing high levels of sexual performance through old age.

Recently Clyde E. Martin, PhD, of the Gerontology Research Center in Baltimore, reported his own studies confirming that. He interviewed 451 men between 45 and 84 years old. His findings: "The results clearly suggest that respondents tended to maintain relatively higher levels of sexual activity over many years of their lives."

Those who were active in their youth stayed active; those who were not failed to maintain an active sex life in old age.

Obviously that is partly hereditary. But, as Dr. Masters suggests, sexual activity itself seems to contribute to a continuing active sex life in old age. Adds Dr. Martin, "Both mechanisms (hereditary and sexual activity) undoubtedly contribute to the maintenance of individual differences."

That the sex act is effective in maintaining capacity throughout life is explainable at least in part through its influence on testosterone levels. There is no question that in most men sexual stimulation increases the amount of testosterone in the blood. In most men and all animals those increased levels stimulate erotic interest and drive unless the intellect overrides the normal biological response. Thus there is more than minimal validity in the cliché, "Use it or lose it."

19

Nutrition and the Testes

Electron planets orbiting their suns at fantastic speeds; chemical oceans compressing eons of decay and oxidation into hours; birth, death, rebirth of cells by the untold millions. Ask any of those cells or the countless billions of bacteria that are born, live, and die in or on us, and they will explain that the human body in which they dwell is not merely a planet but an entire universe. Vast numbers of systems function continuously with such complexity of interactions that some even today are beyond our comprehension. Nothing in our own universe is more complex than the body's chemistry, whereby it maintains an ideal homeostasis (the tendency to keep the internal environment stable and harmonious).

Without that balance, no organ, including the testes, could function properly. Every last cell of the gonads maintains optimal functioning only when a very specific set of requirements are met. Temperature is one. Even more crucial is the availability of certain nutrients.

A fraction of much that a man eats goes to maintaining the size, shape, and function of his testicles, and without that nourishment the glands would atrophy. Beyond gulping the food down, most of us never give it a conscious thought. Yet before the food reaches our mouths, our bodies embark upon their single most complex undertaking—the processing of what we eat. The very sight or smell of food stimulates us to salivate. Teeth and saliva are the first to attack food substances and initiate the digestive process. In the stomach hydrochloric acid takes over, disassembling foods into the basic materials from which they were constructed. The blood absorbs these food chemicals and carries them to the billions upon billions of cells throughout the body. Some nutrients are required by all cells—protein, glucose, certain vitamins, and minerals. Others are needed only by cells of certain tissues.

The cell itself performs the miracle of utilizing the decomposed food substances. Although each cell is invisibly small and the working particles within the cell much smaller yet, these tiny factories utilize enzymes and hormones to create and excrete the same and other enzymes and hormones, to repair and strengthen their cell walls and create new cells—in short, to maintain all the body's functions.

Each cell is like a factory to which the blood brings raw lumber. Some workmen use it to repair the factory roof and worn floorboards. Others carry some of the raw material to the furnace which generates the heat and energy needed to run the factory's equipment. Still other workers process the lumber, creating planks that can be used to build more factories. Additional laborers extract from the lumber certain chemicals, some of which are used in the factory's own operation. Other chemicals are shipped out (into the blood) to meet the needs of other factories.

Cell factories work in groups and form specific tissues—testicles, kidney, heart, brain, and such. There are significant differences among cells. A liver cell, for instance, looks and functions much differently from a muscle cell. The two also have differing nutrient requirements for the same reason that a plastics factory would find useless the wool required by a knitting mill.

That is an important point, for it explains why certain cells (and the organs they compose) can suffer nutritional deficiencies so radical that the organ can no longer function while the rest of the body remains relatively healthy. We know, for example, that the mucous membranes have a heavy vitamin A requirement, that muscle cells need protein, that the liver needs the B complex, and that the brain needs large amounts of oxygen and glucose.

The sex organs are no exception. As long ago as 1889, researchers discovered that the testes of pigeons wasted away when they were not fed adequately. The testes are particularly sensitive to malnutrition. According to Dr. Thaddeus Mann, "Quite often a marked decrease in the growth rate and secretory activity of male accessory organs which follows on even a small degree of underfeeding becomes obvious earlier than regression changes in other organs of the body." Thus even a minor nutritional deficiency, unrecognizable in muscle tissue or liver, may still significantly affect the size and function of the testes.

Researchers at the Ian Clunies Ross Animal Research Laboratory in New South Wales, Australia, recently showed precisely what happens to the testes during malnutrition. For their study they used twelve rams, six well-fed, six on a protein/calorie restricted diet. After three months there was no question which sheep were being underfed. They had less than 12 percent body fat as compared to the well-fed groups' 25 to 28 percent. Predictably, the testes of the well-fed rams were larger. It was the degree of difference that was surprising. The testes of the malnourished rams weighed only .27 percent of their total body weight, while those of the well-fed rams weighed .38 percent, a relative difference of more than 25 percent. Although other organs in the underfed rams were smaller than in the control animals, the reduction remained stable in proportion to the total reduced body weight. Even when compared to other endocrine glands, only the testes lost more than the expected proportion of weight.

There were other changes, too. Since the testes had become smaller, it was not surprising that blood flow through them was reduced. But a careful investigation revealed that even on a unit weight basis the testes cells were not being exposed to the same amount of blood as that of well-nourished rams.

The combination of less testis bulk to produce testosterone and dramatically reduced blood flow to absorb the hormone argues that nutritional deficiency would produce markedly reduced testosterone levels. In fact, that is precisely the case. The well-fed rams had eight times as much testosterone as did the malnourished animals. The nutritionally deficient rams had far fewer interstitial cells, wherein testosterone is manufactured, and those they did have were less distinct and presumably less healthy.

The underfed animals had significantly smaller and less healthy seminiferous tubules to produce sperm. Many were found to be degenerating, and these rams produced far less sperm than healthy ones.

Undoubtedly, testicular atrophy is a valuable survival factor for both the individual and the species. A serious, prolonged food shortage produces malnutrition, and that causes rapid degeneration of the testes and reduced sperm production. The likelihood of more offspring to compete for the limited food supply is reduced. As a secondary precaution the testes produce less testosterone, which promptly decreases the sex drive among animals. That usually has the pronounced effect of curtailing reproduction. In cases where young are still conceived, some species simply consider them an additional source of food.

The biological process apparently functions as well in man as in animals. Many studies show that both sperm production and sex drive significantly decrease in men during famine as well as experimental undernutrition. Why, then, do we have a world full of nations suffering starvation while continuing to overpopulate prodigiously?

The answer once again is that man alone has an intellectual as well as a physiological sex drive. Unlike other animals, he need not wait for biological events, including the accumulation of seminal fluid and the female estrus, to stimulate his eroticism. At any moment he chooses to escape boredom or assure himself of his masculinity, he may self-stimulate. He has the advantage of his intellect—his capacity to fantasize—and continual erotic experiences not only stimulate even malnourished testes to function to some degree, but help to assure eventual conception even when sperm production is low.

The rams were deprived of two major nutrients—proteins and

calories. The deficiencies were radical, not the kind anyone in a modern society is likely to suffer. The exceptions are people who, by following extreme or faddist diets, literally starve themselves. That is common enough to have its own medical name, anorexia nervosa. Often it is a symptom of emotional problems. In a typical case the victim, most commonly a high school girl, may be twenty or thirty pounds below her ideal weight. Yet she is convinced she is fat and adheres to a starvation diet. Occasionally she dies. Almost inevitably her physical maturation will be arrested. She will not develop breasts, normal pubic hair, or the body shape of a woman. Her menstrual cycle will cease. A boy will have the same arrested sex development. In both the male and the female the body immediately sets to work, blocking the function of the organs responsible for producing more mouths to feed.

No one in this country is likely to suffer a significant deficiency of either protein or calories, but the testes need other nutrients, too—vitamins and minerals—and there *is* evidence that subclinical deficiencies of some of these nutrients are not at all rare. Nationwide studies by the federal government show that a

PERCENTAGE OF MEN AND WOMEN 30-60 YEARS OF AGE FROM ALL SECTIONS OF THE UNITED STATES WHO ATE LESS THAN TWO-THIRDS OF THE R.D.A. OF VARIOUS NUTRIENTS.

	Women	Men
Protein	10	5
Iron	18	12
Thiamine	20	15
Riboflavin	30	10
Niacin	20	9
Vitamin A	45	20
Ascorbic Acid	35	35
Calcium	60	30

significant percentage of the population, regardless of age or economic status, survives on diets containing one third or less of the recommended daily allowances. Regarding protein, 5 percent of the men and 10 percent of the women surveyed fit into that category. But as many as 30 percent of the men and 60 percent of the women receive one third or less of the calcium they need. Similar shortages exist in iron, thiamine, riboflavin, niacin, vitamin A, and ascorbic acid.

Precisely those nutrients that are most often lacking are the ones essential to the healthy, normal functioning of the testes. For example, according to the survey by the federal government, one man out of five eats a diet providing not more than two thirds of the amount of vitamin A he needs. Yet Dr. Isobel W. Jennings, pathologist at the University of Cambridge, England, explains in her recent book, *Vitamins in Endocrine Metabolism*, "Advanced A-deficiency in the male rat is equivalent virtually to chemical castration and is associated with degenerative changes in the germinal epithelium of the testis (the tissue covering the testis within the scrotum) and the production of abnormal spermatozoa." Adds Dr. Jennings, "A-deficiency interferes with the synthesis or release of androgens, and not with the state of receptivity of the target cells."

Another researcher who has spent a good deal of time investigating the need for vitamin A in testicular health is Dr. Birthe Palludan of Copenhagen. Palludan says, "Termination—or a marked reduction—of spermatogenesis as a consequence of the A-avitaminosis (vitamin A deficiency) characterized all findings in the species of animals examined." Palludan was working with boars. "It was determined in these experiments that the administration of vitamin A to an A-avitaminotic boar resulted in complete normalization of the spermatogenesis within three months."

In her experiments Palludan gave some of her boars vitamin A acid. The acid form prevents serious infections from developing, but cannot be utilized by the body to satisfy other requirements of vitamin A, including maintaining healthy testicles. Those other needs must be met with vitamin A alcohol or vitamin A aldehyde.

Once Palludan was sure a vitamin A deficiency was present, (she took liver samples and examined them for stores of the vitamin), she began to weigh the animals' testicles. She reported, "The weight of the testicles (in the vitamin A deficient animals) was found to be much lower in all experimental boars than in their normal littermates; members of the former group were about a third or half the normal weight."

Most recent findings suggest that, depending upon what region of the United States we are talking about, vitamin A stores may be low in 12 to 37 percent of the population.

Since 1950 Americans have been eating 31 pounds less of fresh fruit and 20 pounds less of fresh vegetables each year. That undoubtedly accounts for at least some of the deficiency. Here is what one writer, Mary Beane, writing in *Prevention* (February, 1973), concludes from those facts:

> First, let's calculate the average vitamin A content of all these fruits and vegetables. Do this for an assortment of ten varieties, including those which are rich in vitamin A (e.g., broccoli and apricots) and those which are notably lacking in vitamin A (e.g., pears and beets), and you discover that a typical pound of these foods contains slightly less than 5,000 units of vitamin A. Now this is just about the amount which government nutrition publications say we need every day in order to avoid vitamin A deficiency. Now, multiply this deficit by 51 pounds of fruits and vegetables which we aren't eating, and you get an annual deficit of over 225,000 units of vitamin A, or 51 days' worth of vitamin A intake!

Another cause of vitamin A deficiency is disease or infection. It is now known that repeated infections, particularly those involving diarrhea, can drain vitamin A from the body. High fever causes a significant drop in vitamin A levels in the blood, and even physical activity has that effect.

In some cases what might be considered outrageously high doses of the vitamin are essential. Experiments by Dr. H. M. Russell at the University of Chicago Pritzker School of Medicine with five cases of celiac sprue and regional enteritis demonstrated that. Each patient was only subclinically deficient in vitamin A, which means that no frank symptoms of the deficiency were obvious. Yet although the recommended daily allowance for vitamin A is 5,000 IUs, 50,000 to 60,000 units were administered daily for four weeks before normal vitamin A levels were reached.

Nine to fifteen percent of the men the government studied suffered a significant deficiency of at least one factor in the vitamin B complex—thiamine, riboflavin, or niacin. Studies spanning a period of more than forty years show that a vitamin B deficient diet rapidly produces a sharp decline in the genital functions of animals.

Another vitamin that plays a major role in testicular health is vitamin E. In fact, medical texts occasionally refer to it as the antisterility vitamin. In animals vitamin E deficiency leads to deterioration of seminiferous tubules—usually within three months. If the animals are kept on vitamin E deficient diets for six to nine months, they will become completely and irreversibly sterile.

If the deficiency is recognized and treated before it progresses to complete infertility, a cure is possible. Dr. Evan Shute, one of the nation's best-known authorities on vitamin E, has reported on twenty men with very low sperm production who showed increases to normal following vitamin E therapy. Those whose sperm were dead began producing live sperm. Several of these men impregnated their wives within a few months of beginning vitamin E therapy.

Another nutrient that seems to be particularly essential to the genital organs is not a vitamin but a mineral—zinc. Today the role zinc plays in the growth, health, and function of genital organs is receiving much attention. Yet the original research, long ignored, is more than half a century old.

Adult men with infantile sex organs can sometimes be cured through zinc supplementation. One of the first to prove that was Dr. Hossain A. Ronaghy, associate professor of medicine at Pahlavi University School of Medicine in Shiraz, Iran. Dr. Ronaghy learned that at least 187 twenty-year-old men had been exempted from military service in the Iranian Army after medical examination because of inadequate physical maturation. As a group the men were 20 percent lower in height and 45 percent lower in weight than normal. Each of them had low zinc concentration in plasma, hair, and red blood cells—the most reliable sites for measuring zinc concentration. Sexually their development was that of prepubertal children.

Dr. Ronaghy persuaded fifteen of the undeveloped men to live for six months or more in a village near the medical shcool where he worked and to follow a basic diet, which included 20 to 30 mg of zinc daily (nutritionists believe about 12 mg per day is needed to meet the needs of average healthy adults).

The men were divided into two groups. One was given an additional 27 mg of zinc daily in a capsule. The second and larger group was given a placebo. Thus any psychological effect that might be produced by the idea of taking a daily nutritional supplement would affect both groups equally.

Within three months virtually all the men on the zinc supplement matured sexually. Their genitals grew to adult proportions. They began to have nocturnal emissions and developed interest in women. While the group on the placebo grew taller, they did not develop sexually.

Six months after the study began, three men in the placebo group were given the zinc capsules instead. In less than two months they began having nocturnal emissions. The implication, though not yet verified, is that zinc is in some way essential to the body's capacity to utilize testosterone. When the mineral is absent, the hormone is unused, and eventually the testes decline in production of it. But the relationship between the mineral and the hormone may be much more complex than that.

Zinc is also apparently of great importance to the prostate. That gland is by far the richest source of zinc in the body. Only when the prostate is cancerous does the zinc level fall. In animals the testes also have shown high zinc concentration.

If testosterone cannot be used without zinc, the reverse also seems to be true. When animals are castrated, significant reduction takes place in zinc uptake. In some cases—and perhaps all—the hormone and mineral seem to work together.

The moral of this story ought to be obvious, but it is important enough to permit the indulgence of repetition. Many of us, bloated by sweet and fatty foods, decide as we reach middle age and beyond that the sedentary life's most obvious achievement is the roll of fat beneath our belts. Logically we should eliminate the excess weight through regular physical activity. Understandably we choose instead a diet—any of an overwhelming number of fad diets that happen to be in fashion at the time.

The result, when adequate nutrition is most essential (in the middle and later years), is a kind of selective starvation. Almost invariably we continue with the tasty (i.e., sweet and fattening) foods, then react in guilt by eliminating less tasty but more nutritional meals. Some people boast of not eating a single meal all day, while ignoring the round-the-clock snacks upon which they gorge themselves.

The importance of an adequate diet really cannot be exaggerated. High protein, low fat foods are daily essentials. They include organ meats such as liver, heart, kidneys, and brain, and fish and poultry.

Vitamin A can be obtained in ample amounts in apricots, apricot nectar, eggs, parsley, and carrots. The best source by far of vitamin E is wheat germ oil. Six tablespoons of it contain 420 mg of the vitamin. Tomato juice and eggs are also good sources of vitamin E. So are most seeds. Zinc is found in large amounts in pineapple juice and eggs. But the greatest source of zinc is seafoods, especially oysters. That fact has undoubtedly given rise to the myth that oysters are an aphrodisiac.

There are no aphrodisiacs—only nutrients without which the testes and other genital organs cannot grow and function optimally. While the professionals argue the details, the public would do well to realize that *most* of the population receives less than an ideal level of some nutrients in its regular diet.

20
Drugs

The corner drugstore is as basic to the American way of life as the automobile. Hardly a home in the country lacks at least some of the patent medicines sold on the shelves of the local pharmacy. Rare is the infant who, within days or weeks of birth, is not treated to at least one, and often a series of drugs. Often it is to his good fortune that the drugs are available. There can be no serious controversy that drugs not only alleviate symptoms but also cure many diseases and save many lives.

Still, at least in part because drugs have been absorbed so thoroughly into our culture and individual lives, we have tended until recent years to hold them in a completely benign light. Dictionary definitions of drugs as "chemical substances which protect or restore health" enhance the attitude. Yet the fact is that all drugs—even certain vitamins when administered in high doses impossible to obtain in food—are toxic. If they do not have the capacity to force a reaction of some type in the body, then they are not drugs. If they *do* produce a reaction, then by definition they have the potential to do harm.

Most drugs produce not one but several reactions in the body—the desired response and one or more side effects. That is one reason the most effective drugs available require a doctor's prescription. Drugs designed for the sinuses may prove hazardous to the kidneys. Blood pressure drugs may affect the liver. Other drugs may harm the eyes. The list of interactions and potential side effects is virtually without end. Doctors and drug manufacturers recognize that fact and, at least in theory, control adverse reactions by publishing warnings and frequently monitoring patients during the course of prescription drug therapy.

Several drugs, by affecting the hypothalamic-pituitary-gonadal axis, interfere with testicular function and testosterone production. Shakespeare recognized the effects of the most common of those drugs when he wrote that alcohol "provokes the desire, but takes away the performance." The same point was asserted less poetically in 1974 by British researchers. They found that men who are occasional social drinkers have decreased testosterone levels following alcohol consumption. (That particular study suggested that men who consume a lot of alcohol on a regular basis, including alcoholics, build a tolerance so that testosterone levels are not significantly affected.)

Actually the reduced testosterone probably plays a minor role in the decreased sexual capacity of the inebriated. The drug's effect upon the central nervous system is probably sufficient in itself to depress sexual response.

Chronic, excessive alcohol intake often depresses testosterone in another way, too. It damages the liver, causing cirrhosis. The malfunctioning liver produces excess sex hormone binding globulin, which, as we have seen, binds preferentially with testosterone. Additional interstitial cell-stimulating hormone is released in the pituitary, but in amounts insufficient to raise testosterone levels to normal. As a result, hypogonadism and gynecomastia are common developments in alcoholics.

Tranquilizers, too, often depress testosterone levels. One example is phenobarbital, prescribed as a sleeping pill and sedative. It also accelerates the metabolism of testosterone. The result is like shooting off the shotgun before the ducks come into view; there is no ammunition when it is needed.

Chronic use of tranquilizers such as phenobarbital, chlorpromazine, and such over long periods can have a profound negative effect on male sexuality precisely because testosterone is too rapidly metabolized and cleared from the system. A study at the University of Missouri Medical Center showed that the testes of animals subjected to the drug failed to produce typical amounts of testosterone. What's more, only 39.9 percent of the sperm they produced were live, as compared to more than 63 percent in a control group. Other sex organs were also affected. The seminal vesicles decreased in weight by more than 18 percent, and the prostate by 17 percent. Says the leading researcher, Mostafa Fahim, PhD, "Drug (phenobarbital) treatment alone produces changes in male accessory (sex) organs similar to those seen in sexually mature castrate (rats) three days after operation."

Even common over-the-counter preparations interfere with testosterone production. The most widely used include aspirin, phenacetin, and similar nonprescription pain relievers. Eldon Boyd, MD, of Kingston, Ontario, first became interested in the possible link between these drugs and sexuality when he realized that among those of his patients taking from twenty-five to over a hundred of these tablets per day for five to ten years, most were childless. To test the theory that the drugs were related to infertility, Dr. Boyd administered high doses of them to male rats. Each of the animals lost weight on the heavy drug regimen—an average of 15 percent. But their testicular weight dropped 52 percent for phenacetin and 60 percent for acetaminophen. Again the testes seemed to respond more rapidly than the rest of the body to the chemical upset the drug produced. The body does not know how to interpret the internal disruption of homeostasis, but does recognize it as an abnormality (whether or not it is to work to our benefit). The immediate reaction is to lessen the likelihood of procreation and the stresses it may entail on both the individual and the species.

Microscopic examination shows that spermatogenesis is impaired by any radical reduction in testes weight. Attempts to breed the drugged animals with normal females showed the males had a much higher than normal sterility rate. After two months' administration of one of the drugs, phenacetin, 63 percent of the rats were sterile; after three months, the figure reached 72 percent.

Some types of general anesthesia used in surgery have been shown to reduce testosterone levels significantly. In a study involving seventy men between nineteen and sixty-one years of age, researchers have found that nitrous oxide, oxygen, and halothane used in combination caused an 80 percent drop in testosterone levels within two days following surgery. Apparently the hypothalamus recognized the testosterone deficiency and signaled the pituitary, which released gonadotrophins in large quantities to stimulate the testes to produce more hormone. Yet, for at least a week following the surgery, the testes failed to respond.

No one is quite sure just how the anesthesia affects the testes. One theory is that the adrenal glands interpret the unnatural presence of gases in the blood and the unconsciousness they produce as an emergency situation and deal with it by secreting large amounts of cortisone and adrenocorticotrophin (ACTH) into the blood. These hormones are known to be testosterone antagonists and may severely hinder testicular function.

These are only a few of the numerous drugs which affect testosterone levels. Others include those which control blood pressure and some used to prevent gout. Obviously, estrogen-containing substances are antiandrogenic. So are the very popular corticosteroids such as cortisone and ACTH prescribed (far too frequently) for allergies and inflammatory disorders such as arthritis and rheumatism.

Except for relatively few cases, the influence drugs have on testosterone production has not been investigated. Thus even the family doctor with the assistance of drug package inserts, medical reports, and his trusty copy of *Physician's Desk Reference* will be unable to answer with authority questions about a drug's effect on male hormone levels. Certainly at least some cases of waning sexual capacity, musculature, endurance, and overall well-being commonly associated with aging are the result of decreased testosterone levels caused by chronic use of antiandrogenic drugs. Often there is no recourse. Most people suffering severe arthritic pain, for example, would gladly accept reduced testosterone levels in exchange for relief through corticosteroids. Yet that decision should rest as much with the patient as with the physician. Today virtually no patients are told of these potential side effects, frequently because the doctors themselves are not aware of them.

What's more, there is convincing evidence that most drugs are prescribed far more regularly than necessary. To continue with the same example, most research still shows that ordinary aspirin remains the most effective therapy for rheumatic and arthritic pain, and that the corticosteroids with their numerous and sometimes very serious side effects should be reserved for a small minority of cases.

Particularly for the older man concerned with a sense of deteriorating manhood, one of the first areas of suspicion might be his medicine cabinet. Sometimes drug-taking, particularly involving the over-the-counter preparations, becomes habitual rather than essential to well-being. Somehow we have evolved into the "placebo generation," a people who find a sense of security and comfort in swallowing vitamins, aspirins, amphetamines, barbiturates, syrups, tablets, capsules, and lozenges, whether or not they provide an objective benefit.

We simply do not need the awesome quantity of drugs we consume. Not rarely we would be healthier without them, and occasionally more manly.

21

Ribot and Quid—A Summary

He pioneered the basic ideas for the theory of relativity, invented differential calculus, and proposed the construction of a universal language for science, symbolic logic. He is generally recognized as the most versatile and brilliant mind of the seventeenth century. Yet, Gottfried Leibniz is remembered today, disparagingly, for his insistence that "this is the best of all possible worlds."

It was a theistic attitude which Voltaire effectively ridiculed. The ordinary twentieth-century man has *experienced* miracles which even the mind of Leibniz could hardly have imagined. We have seen some diseases, once the torturous killers of hordes, virtually abolished. We have learned to treat the insane as ill humans rather than demon-possessed servants of Satan. We have instituted welfare programs to help the needy, and mission stations and hospitals in foreign lands. Certainly we have made the world a far better place than it was when Leibniz made his famous statement.

Then again, although this century is only about three quarters through, we have already destroyed through war more people than in any century of the world's history. We have seen through riots and assassinations, and bombings and brutality of all sorts, intolerance no less abhorrent (and perhaps more so) than in

Leibniz's day. The philosopher urged a unification of Protestant and Catholic faiths, but today the two faiths remain at war. He sought a universal pooling of knowledge and language; yet nations remain decidedly separate and competitive.

Relieved of its theological trappings, Leibniz's philosophy may have been every bit as brilliant as his mathematics, for he seemed to be making a simple empiric observation about the nature of the world. There are certain factors (we call them laws of nature) governing the universe. Some have to do with gravity, centrifugal force, inertia. Moreover, there are the inviolate laws of biology and the equally inviolate laws of psychobiology. We have conquered killer diseases not by spurning natural laws and functions, but precisely the opposite: We have found ways to utilize natural processes to establish a new homeostasis more to our liking.

There is probably no case in man's history where he has disregarded any fundamental principle upon which the world runs—whether physical, biological, or psychological—to his own betterment. Rather, through such disregard he has stumbled perilously close to the brink of environmental disaster, embraced the chemical implements of abuse to his own body, and won for himself the distinction of being the only animal on earth to take his own life in preference to suffering emotional conflict.

Much can be changed, but the laws are inflexible. Concerning them, we are living not in the best but the *only* possible world. Changes can be made, and must be, but only a fool would conclude that by slaying the goose he could succeed in gathering the greater quantity of golden eggs.

We have been particularly concerned in this book with those laws of nature governing the development of manhood. We have found that a man does not just happen. On the contrary, the natural progression of a zygote is to develop as a female, and only when an additional event takes place, probably stimulated by the chromosomes, do the gonads develop into testes producing hormones which masculinize the embryo. There are comparatively few risks to the sexual development of the female. With some few exceptions the sexually ambiguous infant is a male whose development ceased at some point along the path toward what we generally recognize as "complete" masculinity.

When the man-child is born he is different from the woman-child in a way much more profound than penises and vaginas can demonstrate. Every last cell of his body is different—those that compose his hair, his brain, his heart, his muscle, and the composition of his bone. He is the product of the testosterone that permeates him.

It is not his will that makes him thus. Many a transsexual, desiring to appear feminine, has cursed his large bones and bulging muscle. Usually castration can remove the masculinizing influence and estrogens can inspire a feminizing one. It is another example of obeisance to the natural laws governing masculinity and femininity.

The masculine brain, like that of the burro and rabbit, produces some less than desirable behavioral traits. One is aggressiveness, which enabled primitive man, relatively weak, slow-moving, and defenseless for his size, to conquer his enemies, and his environment, and to establish against inconceivable odds the dominance of the human species throughout the world. Human male aggressiveness is today as cold and savage as it ever was, whether it is displayed on Madison Avenue or in the boxing ring at Madison Square Garden. There is not the slightest indication that ten thousand years of civilization have reduced his aggression one iota. It has merely, in most cases, channeled it in a less destructive direction.

As a gender the female has never even remotely approached the level of aggressiveness which males daily exhibit. Boys fight for pleasure, even in their Sunday clothes, and even when they realize the punishment will be severe. Girls avoid fighting whether or not they have been taught to do so, even when boys taunt them, and even when it is more than reasonable and socially acceptable for them to fight.

The current vogue is to attribute behavioral differences such as aggressiveness to the child's upbringing. The argument is that girls encouraged from birth to be rough-and-tumble will be so, and boys reared to be effeminate will develop in that way. Some widely respected authorities hold that view, and the reason it is difficult to refute is that, like all responsible theories, there is some truth to it. Certainly we absorb much of our personality—the way we walk, speak, and look at life, religion, and politics—from those we live with. A girl learns how a woman acts by observing her mother. And a boy learns how to be a man by subconsciously imitating his father. Certainly some of our sex role behavior is learned.

But all the academic theories notwithstanding, gender-related behavior is much more basic than patterns of speech, movement, and even religious thinking. As we grow into adolescence, we may observe that certain aspects of our speech are not acceptable among educated people. With some effort we change them. We may learn to stop swaggering, strutting, or bouncing if people ridicule us for it, or we find it is not the way most people walk. We may ponder our parents' religion, determine that we do not believe as we were taught, convert to another religion, or become atheists. But we almost *never* change our basic sex-related behavior patterns.

Men who are active and aggressive by nature can playact at passiveness, but they cannot become truly passive. In fact, many cannot even playact—the frustration involved in pretending to relax is intolerable to them. A man with normal heterosexual drives and compulsions could not be conditioned to be content as an active and exclusive homosexual. The reverse is also true.

The evidence for this is overwhelming. Homosexual men testify to recognizing erotic attraction to other men during the first decade of their lives. Some have gone through almost torturous negative conditioning, tolerating violent electric shock and other punishment in order to change their sexual drive. Such methods often fail. Child molesters, rapists, and exhibitionists are jailed time and again and treated through psychoanalysis and other forms of psychiatry—to no avail. Desperately some request castration or lobotomy. It is obvious in the extreme that male sexual compulsion, like aggression, is determined through the natural laws determining our psychobiology, in part the product of the presence or absence of testosterone.

Some individuals entertain the myth that society will eventually achieve a unisex of sorts in which the male and female will be not only equal but, in every sense except the physical, synonymous. The one exception would be that of reproductive physiology, and some theories propose that even that difference may be superfluous once human life can be created in the test tube. Females will be trained from birth to be as aggressive, competitive, and athletic as men. Men will be exposed to domesticity and will learn to care for children with tenderness and patience. And everyone will live happily ever after.

The man incised the belly of the goose, but to his amazement no avalanche of golden eggs ensued. There was not, in fact, a single egg, not the tiniest one—only a dead goose.

Whether or not a psycho-unisexual society would have a place in an ideal world is an interesting question, one that could undoubtedly provide endless debate along with other hypothetical time killers such as the number of angels which could fit on the head of a pin. But we are talking about *practical* things now, the best of all *possible* worlds. Psychounisex is simply not possible.

To return to an earlier theme: For all the verbosity surrounding it, male sexuality is a fragile and tentative thing. Under ideal circumstances the urge to copulate becomes an unbridled compulsion. Yet hunger, thirst, anxiety, fear, grief, elation, pain—any number of factors—can easily take precedence over the male's temperamental sex drive. In her book, *The New Sex Therapy*, psychiatrist and sex therapist Helen Singer Kaplan, MD, PhD, of Cornell University College of Medicine, summarizes male sexual sensitivity as evidenced in his testosterone levels:

> The psychological state of a person influences his androgen level, which tends to fluctuate rather markedly in response to psychic and sexual stimuli. Studies of male humans and lower primates under various conditions suggest the following relationships between male testosterone secretion and experience. Sexually attractive opportunities, stimulation, and activity tend to be associated with an increase of the blood testosterone level. Depression, defeat, and humiliation, such as, for example, loss of a female to another male or defeat in other adversary situations, are

associated with a dramatically lowered testosterone level; chronic inescapable stress, such as experienced during officer candidate training, is also associated with a significantly lowered androgen level.

In doing sexual therapy one is sensitive to such ecologic elements and assesses the nature of the patient's situation in formulating the problem. Thus, when an impotent man is under a great deal of stress, such as during a difficult business crisis or after a destructive divorce, etc., or when he seems to be suffering from depression, it is usually wise to postpone sexual therapy for his impotence or low libido until emotional stability has been regained.

Ribot and Quid could have coauthored a novel, so dramatic were their short lives, had they been humans rather than monkeys. Nothing unique occurred during their childhood or adolescent years. The story begins in early adulthood when, through an act of God (in this case researcher Robert Rose), both suddenly found themselves smack in the middle of a harem.

Ribot was a rather shy fellow, and for the better part of a day after being transferred to the new environment, his testosterone level dropped from more than 1,000 nanograms per 100 ml of plasma to less than 500. But he was still a perfectly normal monkey, and it did not take him long to realize that he was surrounded by a group of giggling, crouching, sexually submissive, and eager females. In just over a week his testosterone level soared to almost 2,000. Under its influence he became very active sexually.

Then, after two weeks, Dr. Rose removed Ribot from the females. His testosterone level promptly fell to the baseline of about 1,000.

Quid's experience was similar, except that he was not nearly as shy as Ribot. Hardly had he been introduced to his own harem when his testosterone levels soared from about 750 to approximately 1,600, and then continued on up to almost 2,000. When he was removed from the females, his plasma androgen returned to base levels.

The next development in the lives of Ribot and Quid was brutal in the extreme. One morning Dr. Rose tossed each of them into a neighborhood bossed by a gang of hoodlum monkeys. For two weeks they were taunted, beaten, and bullied by the others. They spent days and nights cowering alone in a corner of the yard, constantly fearful of attack.

Unlike others in the experiment, Ribot and Quid were fortunate in not needing any sutures. But their emotional traumas could have rivaled anything in *West Side Story*. One result was that their testosterone levels plunged—in Quid's case to about half baseline, and in shy Ribot's to less than one fourth of normal.

In the best Hollywood tradition it is a story of love gained, lost, and regained. A few weeks after their defeat, so dramatic that it was a virtual hormonal castration, Dr. Rose reintroduced Ribot and Quid to their respective harems. Both shot back to their 2,000 mark almost immediately, but this time it was Ribot who responded first. All of which proves that the right females can do wonders even for the most timid man or monkey.

Actually, Ribot and Quid prove a good deal more than that. At the risk of offending the few who may not thus far have been offended, let us state bluntly, as does C. A. Tripp in his book, *The Homosexual Matrix*, that the subjection of the female to the male, has always been essential to functional sexuality. It is this response to the male's biologically inspired dominance that maintains the male's testosterone levels and sexual capacity. In animals this is always true; in man the intellect dilutes and taints the natural biological response but does not basically alter it.

Our society today entertains a fascinating paradox. (Now paradoxes are not necessarily undesirable or even illogical, but they do strongly recommend investigation, for they may harbor contradiction, and contradiction *is* illogical.) On the one hand, we are finally moving toward respect for that which is ecological, a wise and long-needed appreciation for the ambiance of nature, a philosophy of cooperation with the laws that govern this only possible world. On the other hand, a small vocal minority advocate spurning the laws governing our psychobiology. One of the most striking examples is the trend toward coeducational physical activities and sports. Says Derik H. Miller, MD, professor of psychiatry at the University of Michigan Medical Center:

> This is probably the most insensitive effort ever perpetrated by the bureaucracy in this field as it ignores the psychological needs of both boys and girls.
>
> Girls have a greater need for privacy than boys, particularly in puberty, and may have great sensitivity about forced exposure, particularly during activities such as swimming and physical education. . . .
>
> Psychology of the pubertal male is particularly being ignored. Prior to puberty, males have no particular problem in relating to girls on equal terms. The male is probably slightly bigger than the same age girl and so feels secure in relation to her physically. The three years of puberty is the only time in a boy's life that he is likely to experience himself as smaller than the equivalent age girl. Pubescent boys are also less effective intellectually and emotionally than girls. The pubescent male is threatened by close proximity of females of the same age. Regulations which insist that pubertal boys and girls join together in sports activities are psychologically inappropriate. The likelihood is that either boys will refuse to take part, or behave with inappropriate aggression. Future tenderness between the sexes is not likely to be reinforced.

Some authorities view what is generally termed equality among the sexes with a degree of trepidation. Says Richard A. Gardner, MD, of Columbia University College of Physicians and Surgeons, "A new generation of men will have to be developed who have the ego-strength to relate to a woman on the egalitarian basis. If such men do not develop, the new liberated, educated, and skilled woman will find herself with a new problem—that of not having suitable mates available."

Nonetheless, the women's liberation movement is far more beneficial than it is disastrous for three reasons. First is the obvious: Women, like coal miners at the turn of the century, migrant workers today, and artists in almost all ages and all cultures, receive neither the respect nor recompense they deserve for the work they do, whether in the home or community. Nor have they been free to apply for some jobs at which certain of them may have been more skilled than male applicants. (The discrimination also applied to men, who were until recently rarely considered as secretaries, stewards on airlines, telephone operators, and such.) Women followed the example of male factory workers before them, organized, and forced upon their employers in many cases equal compensation for equal work. Inequities still exist and need to be actively condemned and eliminated.

The second benefit, a more clearly defined dichotomy between the sexes, will not be so promptly forthcoming, for it will depend in part on the evolutionary development of both men and women. Make no mistake. Nature is clearly on the side of the differentiation of the sexes. She had the amoeba, but moved on to sexual reproduction and to the development of maleness, and today zealously guards it through sex hormone binding globulin, which, according to Dr. David Anderson, "represents an important mechanism for the maintenance of differentiation of secondary sexual characteristics in the human adult."

Certainly some, perhaps many, men will be intimidated and stressed by aggressive masculine role-playing among a minority of females in our society. Some of these men will obviously avoid those women as Dr. Gardner suggests they may. A fraction of those, apparently a growing minority, will find homosexual relationships sufficiently satisfying and far less stressful, and so completely avoid women. *In general*, heterosexual couplings will be sought only by men with very high testosterone—i.e., aggression/sexual compulsion—levels. The liberated women will find these men particularly offensive. Only the passive, submissive, highly estrogenic woman will be attracted to them. Copulations will produce highly androgenized boys and highly estrogenized girls, thus reinforcing sexual differentiation.

There is a third advantage to any movement that questions the basic differences between male and female: it leads to clearer insight into what is truly psychobiological and what has been foisted upon us as role-playing conformity to society. For example, we know through animal studies that violence is not at all essential to dominance and aggression, that often the least challenged leaders with the highest testosterone levels control other animals through what seems to be a strength of their "personality," rather than attack and warfare. Masculinity does not preclude tenderness and even what we commonly think of as maternal behavior. In fact, there is evidence that excessive testosterone stimulates tenderness and protective or maternal behavior toward young in male animals. Both boys and girls are undoubtedly taught to role-play a great many traits we generally assume to be psychobiological to the gender. Distinguishing those which are truly such from the societally prescribed ones will provide invaluable relief and benefit to all.

In Reinhold Niebuhr's words: "O God, give us the serenity to accept what cannot be changed, courage to change what should be changed, and wisdom to distinguish the one from the other."

Glossary

ANABOLISM. The process whereby new body tissues are constructed from simple nutrients. Testosterone is essential to the normal anabolic process in man.

ANDROGEN. Any hormone which has a masculinizing effect on the body. Testosterone is by far the most potent.

CATABOLISM. The opposite of anabolism, this is the process whereby body tissue is broken down into simpler substances and either utilized for other needs or excreted as waste.

CHROMATIN. The readily stainable portion of a cell nucleus. It carries the genes of inheritance, and by the chromatin's reaction to staining, a physician can determine the genetic sex of an individual, regardless of physical appearance.

CLIMACTERIC. The change of life that troubles 15 to 35 percent of males in their fifties and is probably related in most cases to decreasing testosterone production.

CRYPTORCHIDISM. Undescended testicles.

EPIDIDYMIS. The small convoluted tubes attached to the top of each testicle. Sperm spend two months traveling through this network, during which time they approach maturity.

ESTROGENS. A group of hormones which produce female characteristics, including estrus, breast development, placement of body fat, and a vaginal environment receptive to sexual activity. The term is analogous to androgens in the male.

FETUS. The potential baby from the fourth month after conception until delivery. Prior to the fourth month, the fetus is referred to as an embryo.

FOLLICLE-STIMULATING HORMONE (FSH). Secreted by the pituitary gland, FSH stimulates the testes to produce sperm cells. In women, FSH stimulates the ovaries to develop and to produce estrogens.

GAMETE. The ovum, or sperm cell, which is capable of uniting to form a zygote, the cell which will normally develop into an embryo.

GONADOTROPHIC HORMONES. Hormones which stimulate the gonads (the testes in men, the ovaries in women) to function and secrete their own hormones.

GONADOTROPHIN-RELEASING HORMONE (GRH). Produced by the hypothalamus, GRH stimulates the pituitary gland to release the hormones which stimulate the testes. The cycle is completed when the testes pour testosterone into the blood. The male hormone reaches the hypothalamus, causing it to cease producing gonadotrophin-releasing hormone.

GYNECOMASTIA. Abnormal breast enlargement.

HORMONE. A chemical secreted by an endocrine gland to control activity of other organs. The term is from the Greek, "I arouse to activity."

HORMONAGEN. A hormone precursor. When activated by an enzyme, it is converted to a hormone.

HUMAN CHORIONIC GONADOTROPHIN (HCG). Made in the placenta, the sac surrounding the fetus, HCG can stimulate the testosterone and sperm production in men, as well as correlative responses in the female. Drug companies extract it from the urine of pregnant women.

HYPOGONADISM. A condition in which the testes are underdeveloped.

HYPOSPADIAS. A condition in which the urethral opening in the male, normally found at the tip of the penis, develops on the underside of the shaft.

HYPOTHALAMIC-PITUITARY-GONADAL AXIS. The relationship between the hypothalamus, pituitary gland and testes referred to above. (See gonadotrophin-releasing hormone.)

INTERSTITIAL CELLS. The cells found in the small gaps or spaces (interstices) which exist between the sperm-producing tubules of the testicular tissue. The interstitial cells produce testosterone. Also called Leydig cells.

INTERSTITIAL CELL-STIMULATING HORMONE (ICSH). This hormone, like FSH, is secreted by the pituitary gland. It stimulates the interstitial cells of the testes to produce testosterone. Sometimes it is referred to as luteinizing hormone.

17-KETOSTEROIDS. Weak androgens and other nonandrogenic hormones, precursors of which are produced by the adrenal glands.

LEYDIG CELLS. (See interstitial cells.)

MICROPHALLIC. Having a very small, almost nonexistent phallus.

PITUITARY GONADOTROPHINS. (See follicle-stimulating hormone and interstitial cell-stimulating hormone.)

PLACEBO. A substance with no medicinal effect but which sometimes renders a cure of many ailments, including sexual impotence, through the power of suggestion.

PREGNENOLONE. A hormone precursor related to cholesterol which the body converts into both male and female hormones.

PROGESTERONE. A female hormone.

PROGESTIN. A precursor to the female hormone, progesterone.

PSYCHOGENIC (or PSYCHIC) IMPOTENCE. Inability to attain or maintain an erection; caused by psychological inhibitions rather than physical ailments.

REBOUND RESPONSE. A phenomenon following discontinuance of testosterone therapy in which the testes resume sperm and testosterone production, sometimes at levels greater than before testosterone therapy was undertaken.

SEX HORMONE BINDING GLOBULIN (SBG). A protein which binds with testosterone in the blood, rendering the hormone incapable of producing its normal function in the male.

STEROIDS. These are fatlike compounds related to alcohol but crystalline. Among the more common steroids in the body are cholesterol, bile acids, and the sex hormones, including testosterone.

Bibliography

"Anabolic Steroids: Doctors Denounce Them, but Athletes Aren't Listening." *Science,* 176 (June 30, 1972),1399–1401.

"Anabolic Steroids of No Value in Improving Athletic Performance." *Journal of the American Medical Association,* 233 (August 4, 1975), 463.

ANDERSON, DAVID C. "Sex Hormone Binding Globulin." *Clinical Endocrinology,* 3 (1974), 69–96.

ARIEL, GIDEON. *The Effect of Anabolic Steroids on Reflex Components and Skeletal Muscle Contractile Force.* Boston: University of Massachusetts, Department of Exercise Science, 1972.

"Aversion Therapy Uses Shock to Bar Homosexual Behavior." *Medical World Tribune* (August 9, 1972), 9.

BEANE, MARY. "Better Health Begins with Vitamin A." *Prevention* (February 1973), 109–24.

"Benign Prostate Hypertrophy Aided by Progesterones." *Modern Medicine* (March 9, 1970), 157.

BENJAMIN, HARRY, MD. *The Transsexual Phenomenon.* New York: Julian Press, 1966.

BERGER, ROBERT A., MD, et al. "Failure of Topical Testosterone in Male-Pattern Alopecia." *Journal of the American Medical Association,* 204 (May 6, 1968), 451 52.

BRAIM, REGINALD T. *Skin Diseases.* Chicago: Regnery, 1955.

BRANDES, DAVID. *Male Accessory Sex Organs.* New York: Academic Press, 1974.

British Journal of Nutrition, 27 (March 1972).
BRODIE, H. KEITH, et al. "Plasma Testosterone Levels in Heterosexual and Homosexual Men." *American Journal of Psychiatry*, 131 (January 1974), 81-83.
BUTLER, ROBERT N. "Sexual Advice to the Aging Male." *Medical Aspects of Human Sexuality* (September 1975), 155-56.
CASHMAN, JOHN. *The LSD Story*. Greenwich, Connecticut: Fawcett Publications, 1966.
"Climacteric." *Medical World News* (June 28, 1974), 44.
CURETON, THOMAS. *The Physiological Effects of Exercise Programs on Adults*. Springfield, Illinois: Charles C. Thomas Press, 1971.
DAHL, DOUGLAS S., MD. "Obstructing Prostatic Calculi in a Eunuch." *Journal of the American Medical Association*, Vol. 212, No. 4 (April 27, 1970), 621-22.
DARBY, CARYL W., et al. "Testosterone Cream: Use or Abuse?" *The Lancet* (September 7, 1974), 598.
DAVIDSON, E. A. "Structure and Metabolism of Skin Polysaccharides." In *Advances in Biology of Skin Aging*, Vol. 6, ed. William Montagna. New York: Pergamon, 1965.
DE KRUIF, PAUL. *The Male Hormone*. New York: Harcourt, Brace & Co., 1945.
DOERING, CHARLES H., et al. "A Cycle of Plasma Testosterone in the Human Male." *Journal of Clinical Endocrinology and Metabolism*, 40 (1975), 492.
DOERR, PETER, MD, et al. "Plasma Testosterone, Estradiol, and Semen Analysis in Male Homosexuals." *Archives of General Psychiatry*, 29 (December 1973), 829-33.
DORNER, G., et al. "Homo- and Hypersexuality in Rats with Hypothalamic Lesions." *Neuroendocrinology*, 4 (1969), 20-24.
ECKSTEIN, GUSTAV. *The Body Has a Head*. New York: Harper & Row, 1969.
EDWARDS, ALLEN. *Erotica Judaica*. New York: Julian Press, 1967.
EDWARDS, D. "Mice: Fighting by Neonatally Androgenized Females." *Science*, 161 (1968), 1027-28.
EHRHARDT, A.A., and J. MONEY, "Progestin-Induced Pseudohermaphroditism: I.O. and Psychosexual Identity in a Study of Ten Girls." *Journal of Sex Research*, III (1967), 83-100.
EIK-NESS, KRISTEN G. *The Androgens of the Testis*. New York: Marcel Dekker, Inc., 1970.

FOX, C. A., et al. "Studies on the Relationship Between Plasma Testosterone Levels and Human Sexual Activity." *Journal of Endocrinology*, 52 (1972), 51–58.

FRIEDMAN, MEYER, MD, and RAY H. ROSENMAN, MD. *Type A Behavior and Your Heart.* New York: Alfred A. Knopf, 1974.

FROIMOVICH, JOSÉ S. "Spermiogron–Response to Testosterone Therapy in Old Men." In *Proceedings of the 7th International Congress of Gerontology,* Vol. 2. Wiener Medizinische Akademie, Wien, Austria, 1965.

FUKUTANI, KEIKO, et al. "Effects of Depot Testosterone Therapy on Serum Levels of Luteinizing Hormone and Follicle-Stimulating Hormone in Patients with Klinefelter's Syndrome and Hypogonadotropic Eunuchoidism." *Journal of Clinical Endocrinology and Metabolism,* 39 (1974), 856–63.

GELLER, JACK, MD, et al. "Therapy with Progestational Agents in Advanced Benign Prostatic Hypertrophy." *Journal of the American Medical Association*, Vol. 210, No. 8. (November 24, 1969), 1421–27.

GLENN, JAMES F., MD. "Microphallneurosis (Small Penis Anxiety Syndrome)." *Journal of the American Medical Association*, Vol. 216, No. 11 (June 14, 1971), 1871.

HAMILTON, J. B. "The Role of Testicular Secretions as Indicated by the Effects of Castration in Man." In *Recent Progress in Hormone Research*, ed. Gregory Pincus, MD, Vol. 3. New York: Academic Press, 1947 50.

HARRISON, RICHARD J., and WILLIAM MONTAGNA. *Man.* New York: Appleton-Century-Crofts, 1969.

"A Hormone Chemistry?" *Medical World News* (November 19, 1971), 15–17.

HOPPNER, et al. *Journal of the Canadian Medical Association* (December 13, 1969).

"Hormones and Elderly Testes." *British Medical Journal* (July 5, 1975), 2–3.

HUFFER, VIRGINIA, MD, et al. "Psychological Studies of Adult Male Patients with Sexual Infantilism Before and After Androgen Therapy." *Annals of Internal Medicine*, Vol. 61, No. 2 (August 1964), 255–68.

IMPERATO-MCGINLEY, JULIANNE, et al. "Steroid 5 of Reductase Deficiency in Man: An Inherited Form of Male Pseudohermaphroditism." *Science,* 186 (December 27, 1974), 1213–15.

INGLEMAN-SUNBERG, A. *Current Problems in Fertility.* New York: Plenum Press, 1971.

JAMES, V. H. T., et al., eds. *The Endocrine Function of the Human Testis,* Vol. 2. New York: Academic Press, 1974.

JONES, JAMES R. "Plasma Testosterone Levels and Female Transsexualism." *Archives of Sexual Behavior,* Vol 2, No. 3 (1973), 251–56.

JULL, J. W., et al. "Hormone Excretion Studies of Males with Gynaecomastia," *British Medical Journal,* 2 (September 26, 1964),797–99.

JULTY, SAM. *Male Sexual Performance.* New York: Grosset & Dunlap, 1975.

KAPLAN, HELEN SINGER, MD, PhD. *The New Sex Therapy.* New York: Brunner Mazel, 1974.

KAYE, HARVEY E., MD. *Male Survival.* New York: Grosset & Dunlap, 1974.

KELLY, HOWARD A., MD. *Cyclopedia of American Medical Biology.* Philadelphia: W. B. Saunders, 1912.

KEMPF, EDWARD J. "The Social and Sexual Behavior of Infrahuman Primates," *Psychoanalytic Review,* 4 (1917), 127–54.

KENT, SAUL. "Impotence: The Facts Versus the Fallacies." *Geriatrics,* Vol. 30, No. 4 (April 1975), 164–71.

KOLODNY, ROBERT, et al. "Plasma Gonadotrophins and Prolactin in Male Homosexuals," *The Lancet* (July 1, 1972), 18–20.

KREUZ, LEO E., MD, Maj. MC, et al. "Assessment of Aggressive Behavior and Plasma Testosterone in a Young Criminal Population." *Psychosomatic Medicine,* Vol. 34, No. 4 (July/August 1972), 321–32.

——— "Suppression of Plasma Testosterone Levels and Psychological Stress." *Archives of General Psychiatry,* 26 (May 1972), 479–82.

KUNTZLEMAN, CHARLES T., ed. *The Physical Fitness Encyclopedia.* Emmaus, Pennsylvania: Rodale Press, 1970.

KUPPERMAN, HERBERT S., MD, PhD, IVEN S. YOUNG, MD, CYNTHIA VAUGHAN, RNMA. *Male Hypogonadism.*

LAMENSDORF, HUGH, MD. "Testosterone Rebound Therapy in the Treatment of Male Infertility." *Fertility and Sterility,* Vol. 26, No. 5 (May 1975), 469–72.

LEVINE, SEYMOUR, and RICHARD F. MULLINS, JR. "Hormonal

Influences on Brain Organization in Infant Rats." *Science*, 152 (June 17, 1966), 1585–92.

——— "Sex Differences in the Brain." *Scientific American*, 214 (1966), 84–90.

LEWINSOHN, RICHARD, MD. *A History of Sexual Customs*. New York: Bell Publishing Co., 1957.

LINDEMAN, BARD. "Cellular Therapy: A Shabby Clinic Offered Rejuvenation but Delivered Death." *Today's Health* (June 1975), 36–41.

LIPSETT, MORTIMER B., MD, et al. "Androgen Metabolis." *Journal of the American Medical Association,* Vol. 190, No. 8 (November 23, 1964), 147–52.

LUNDE, DONALD T., and DAVID A. HAMBURG. "Assessing Effects of Hormones on Aggression." In *Recent Progress in Hormone Research*, ed. E. B. Atwood. Vol. 28, New York: Academic Press, 1972.

LUSCHEN, MARY E., and DAVID M. PIERCE. "Effect of the Menstrual Cycle on Mood and Sexual Arousability." *Journal of Sex Research*, Vol. 8, No. 1 (February 1972), 41–47.

MCGRADY, PAT. *The Savage Cell.* New York: Basic Books, 1964.

MAGUIRE, HENRY C., JR., MD. "Terminal Hair Growth Confined to the Site of Locally Administered Testosterone in the Adult Woman." *Journal of Investigative Dermatology*, Vol. 45, No. 6 (1965), 419–21.

"Male Hormone Production Has Its Ups and Downs." *Medical World News* (March 31, 1967), 30.

MAISEL, ALBERT A. *The Hormone Guest.* New York: Random House, 1965.

MANOSEVITZ, MARTIN. "The Development of Male Homosexuality." *The Journal of Sex Research,* Vol. 8, No. 1 (February 1972), 31–40.

MANTEGAZZA, PAOLO. *The Sexual Relations of Mankind*, translated by Samuel Putnam. New York: Eugenics Publishing Co., 1935.

MASTERS, WILLIAM H., and VIRGINIA E. JOHNSON. *Human Sexual Inadequacy*. Boston: Little, Brown, 1970.

MAZZI, C., et. al. "Gonadotrophins and Plasma Testerone in Senescence, " Vol. II, *The Endocrine Function of the Human Testis,* V.H.T. James, M. Serio, and L. Martini, eds. New York: Academic Press, 1974.

MIRSKY, A. F., et al. "The Influence of Sex Hormones on Social

Behavior in Monkeys." *Journal of Comparative Physiology and Psychology,* 48 (1955), 48.

MONEY, JOHN, and RICHARD R. CLOPPER, JR. "Postpubertal Psychosexual Function in Post-Surgical Male Hypopituitarism." *Journal of Sex Research,* Vol. 11, No. 1 (February 1975), 25–38.

——— "Sexual Dimorphism and Homosexual Gender Identity." *Psychological Bulletin,* Vol. 74, No. 6 (1970), 425–40.

MORGAN, A. F. *Nutritional Status USA 1959.* Agricultural Experimental Station Bulletin, 769, Berkeley, California.

MORRISSEAU, PAUL M. "Viral Prostatitis." *The Journal of Urology,* 103 (June 1970), 103.

NANKIN, HOWARD R., et al. "Daytime Titers of Testosterone LH. Estrone, Estnadiol, and Testosterone-Binding Protein: Acute Effects of LF and LH-Releasing Hormone in Man." *Journal of Clinical Endocrinology and Metabolism,* Vol. 41, No. 2 (1975), 271–81.

NETTER, FRANK H., MD, comp. *The CIBA Collection of Medical Illustrations,* Vol. 4, *Endocrine System and Selected Metabolic Diseases.* Summit, New Jersey: CIBA, 1965.

——— *The CIBA Collection of Medical Illustrations,* Vol. 2, *Reproductive System.* Summit, New Jersey: CIBA, 1954.

NEUMAN, F., et al. "Aspects of Androgen-Dependent Events as Studied by Antiandrogens," Vol. 26. *Recent Progress in Hormone Research,* ed. E. B. Astwood. New York: Academic Press, 1970.

PAPA, CHRISTOPHER M., and ALBERT M. KLIGMAN. "The Effect of Topical Steroids on the Aged Axilla," in *Advances in Biology of Skin Aging,* ed. William Montagna, Vol. 6. New York: Pergamon, 1965.

——— "Stimulation of Hair Growth by Topical Application of Androgens." *Journal of the American Medical Association* Vol. 191, 7 (February 15, 1965), 81–85.

PARKS, GARY A., et al. "Variation in Pituitary-Gonadal Function in Adolescent Male Homosexuals and Heterosexuals." *Journal of Clinical Endocrinology and Metabolism,* 39 (1974), 796.

PASCHKIS, KARL E., MD. *Clinical Endocrinology.* New York: Hoeber-Harper, 1954.

PERSKY, H., et al. "Relationship of Hostility and Testosterone

Production Rate in Normal Young Men." *Psychosomatic Medicine*, 32 (September/October 1970), 553.

——— "Relation of Psychologic Measures of Aggression and Hostility to Testosterone Production in Man." *Psychosomatic Medicine*, Vol. 33, No. 3 (May/June 1971), 265–77.

PINCUS, GREGORY, and KENNETH V. THIMANN, eds. *The Hormones*, Vol. 2. New York: Academic Press, 1950.

PINKE, KARL M., and PETER DOERR. "Age Related Changes and Interrelationships Between Plasma Testosterone Oestradiol and Testosterone-Binding Globulin in Normal Adult Males." *Acta Endocrinologica*, 74 (December 1973), 792–800.

POCHI, PETER E., and JOHN S. STRAUSS. "The Effect of Aging on the Activity of the Sebaceous Gland in Man," Chapter 8, in *Advances in Biology of Skin Aging*, ed. William Montagna, Vol. 6. New York: Pergamon, 1965.

PROUT, GEORGE R., JR., MD. "Response of Men with Advanced Prostatic Carcinoma to Exogenous Administration of Testosterone." *Cancer*, 20 (November 1967), 1871–78.

REITER, TIBERIUS. "Testosterone Implantation: The Method of Choice for Treatment of Testosterone Deficiency." *Journal of the American Geriatrics Society*, Vol. 13, No. 12 (December 1965), 540–50.

RENSBERGER, BOYCE. "Homosexuality Linked to Hormone Level." *New York Times* (November 18, 1971).

RESKO, JOHN A. "Fetal Hormones and Their Effect on the Differentiation of the Central Nervous System in Primates." *Federation Proceedings*, Vol. 34, No. 8 (July 1975), 1650–55.

RIVAROLA, M., et al. "Testosterone Andiostenedione Production." *Journal of Clinical Endocrinology Metabolism* , 26 (November 1966), 1208–18.

ROBINSON, VICTOR, MD. *The Story of Medicine*. New York: The New Home Library, 1931.

ROSE, ROBERT M., et al. "Plasma Testosterone Dominance Rank and Aggressive Behavior in Male Rhesus Monkeys." *Nature*, 231 (June 11, 1971), 366–68.

——— "Androgen Responses to Stress," II. *Psychosomatic Medicine*, Vol. 31, No. 5 (1969), 418–35.

——— "Plasma Testosterone Levels in the Male Rhesus: Influences of Sexual and Social Stimuli." *Science,* 178 (November 10, 1972), 643–65.

ROWLEY M. J., and C. G. HELLER. "The Testosterone Rebound Phenomenon in Treatment of Male Infertility." *Fertility and Sterility,* Vol. 23, No. 7 (July 1972), 498–504.

RUBENS, R. "Further Studies on Leydig Cell Function in Old Age." *Journal of Clinical Endocrinology*, 30 (1974), 40–45.

RUBIN, PHILIP, MD. "Cancer of the Urogenital Tract: Prostatic Cancer." *Journal of the American Medical Association,* Vol. 209, No. 11 (September 15, 1969), 1695–1703.

RUBIN, ROBERT T., et al. "Nocturnal Increase of Plasma Testosterone in Men: Relation to Gonadotropins and Prolactin." *Journal of Clinical Endocrinology and Metabolism,* Vol. 40, No. 6 (1975), 1027–33.

RUEBSAAT, HELMUT J., MD., and RAYMOND HULL. *The Male Climacteric*. New York: Hawthorn Books, 1975.

SAGHIR, MARCEL T. "Homosexuality—II, Sexual Behavior of the Male Homosexual." *Archives of General Psychiatry,* 21 (August 1969), 219–29.

SCHJOTH, A. E. "The Effect of Physical Activity on the Vitamin A Absorption Test." *Scandinavian Journal of Clinical and Laboratory Investigation,* Vol. 17, No. 3 (1965).

SHIPLEY, R. A. "The Gonads and Aging." *Journal of the American Geriatrics Society*, 10 (1962), 26.

SHOEMAKER, TED. "Operation to Relieve Perversion." *Science News*, 97 (January 10, 1970), 50.

SILBER Igal, et al. "The Incidence of Elevated Acid Phosphatase in Prostatic Infarction." *The Journal of Urology*, 103 (June 1970), 765–66.

SMITH, , C. V. M. *The Brain.* New York: Capricorn Books, 1972.

SMITH, KEITH D., et al. "Rapid Oscillations in Plasma Levels of Testosterone, Luteinizing Hormone and Follicle-Stimulating Hormone in Men." *Fertility and Sterility*, Vol. 25, No. 11 (November 1974), 965–75.

SOBOTKA, JOSEPH J., MD "An Evaluation of Afrodex in the Management of Male Impotency: A Double-Blind Crossover Study." *Current Therapeutic Research*, Vol. 11, No. 2 (February 1969), 87–94.

SOLOMON NEIL, MD, PhD, and NATHAN W. SHOCK, PhD. "Nutrition in

the Aged." *Southern Medical Journal*, 62 (December 1969), 1523–28.
"Spermiogram—Response to Testosterone Therapy in Old Men." In *7th International Congress of Gerontology, Biology and Clinical Medicine, Proceedings,* Vienna, Austria, Vol. 2 (June 26 to July 2, 1966), 109–112.
STABLER, TIMOTHY A., PhD, et al. Lecture delivered at the Federation of American Societies for Experimental Biology, Annual Meeting, 1969.
STAMEY, T. A., et al. "Antibacterial Nature of Prostatic Fluid." *Medical Digest* (January 1969), 21.
STARKA, L., et al. "Plasma Testosterone in Male Transsexuals and Homosexuals." *The Journal of Sex Research,* Vol. 11, No. 2 (May 1975), 134-38.
SUTTON, J. R., et al. "Androgen Responses During Physical Exercise." *British Medical Journal,* 1 (1973), 520.
TRIPP, C. A. *The Homosexual Matrix.* New York: McGraw-Hill, 1975.
TURNER, HENRY, MD. *Clinical Use of Testosterone.* Springfield, Illinois: Charles Thomas, 1950.
UDRY, J. RICHARD, and NAOMI M. MORRIS. "Distribution of Coitus in Menstrual Cycle." *Nature*, 220 (November 9, 1968), 593–96.
VEITH, ILZA, PhD. "Intercultural Thoughts on Sexual Mores." *Modern Medicine* (September 20, 1971), 200–6.
VILLE, DOROTHY B., MD. *Human Endocrinology*. Philadelphia: W. B. Saunders Co., 1975.
WESSON, MILEY B., MD. "The Value of Testosterone to Men Past Middle Age." *Journal of the American Geriatrics Society*, 12 (1964), 1149–53.
"Why Is the Brain Male or Female?" *Exerpta.* Emory University (December 1971).
WILLIAMS, ROBERT H., MD, ed. *Testbook of Endocrinology,* 4th ed. Philadelphia: W. B. Saunders Co., 1968.
WILLIAMS, ROGER T. *Biochemical Individuality.* Austin, Texas: University of Texas Press, 1974.
WILSON, ROBERT, MD. *Feminine Forever.* New York: M. Evans, 1966.
WOLSTENHOLME, G. E. W., and MAEVE O'CONNOR. "Ciba Foundation Colloquia on Endocrinology," Vol. 16, *Endocrinology of the Testis.* Boston: Little, Brown and Co., 1967.

Index

Appendix

Since chapter 14 was written, additional studies have added support to the argument that attraction to people of the same sex is a normal development in a given percentage of the population. One of these, authored by Simon LeVay, a neuroscientist with the Salk Institute, appeared in the August, 1991, issue of **Science**, and showed that the hypothalamus, which influences, and perhaps controls, sexual behavior, contains certain cells which, in gay men, are about the same size as those in women--which is half the size of the ones in heterosexual men.

In December of that same year, Michael Bailey and Richard Pillard reported in the **Archives of General Psychiatry** that 52 percent of identical twin brothers--sharing exactly the same genes--were both gay, as 22 percent of fraternal twins, and only 11 percent of unrelated men who had been raised as brothers.

Some spokespersons for the gay community have insisted, in the words of Joyce Hunter, president of the National Lesbian and Gay Health Foundation, that, "in any kind of research one has to examine the ethics and the ramifications." This translates into denying what is clearly a fact scientifically--that at least in some cases homosexuality is genetic--because we don't like what the truth might lead to. But no intelligent person dare participate in such hypocrisy.

The fear is that, if homosexuality is genetic, efforts may someday be made to "correct" this "disease" in the fetal stage. That smacks of hysteria in a day when states have passed gay rights laws, when ten percent of the voting population is widely courted by politicians, and when, even in the Bible Belt, there is a growing tolerance of homosexuals, and laws are being passed against "fag bashing." But apart from all that, it should be beneath the gay community to join the lie for fear of the truth.

These gay leaders argue that the object of desire is "a choice," but anyone who has lusted knows otherwise. It is a **compulsion**, often overwhelming, whether straight or gay. We do not choose; we respond as it is natural and ordained that we respond--ordained by our genes. And we should be proud of that response, whatever it mav be, because it is normal for us. We need not make the ridiculous argument that our sexual passion is merely a choice.

It is, to the core, who we are.